CELEBRATE
YOUR
PREGNANCY

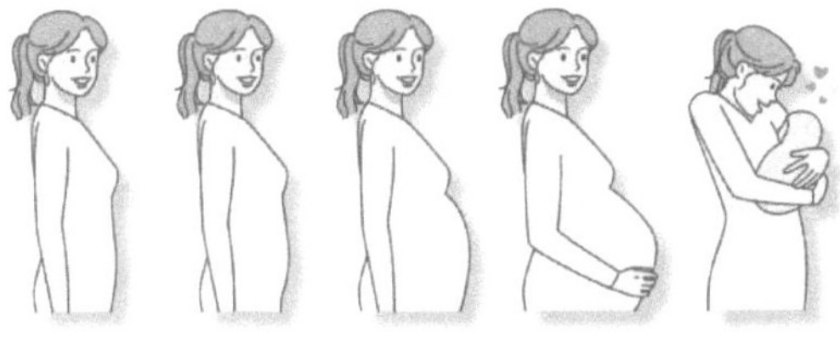

Embrace the Joy of Holding New Life, Conquer Your Emotions &anxieties, Achieve Radiant Well-being and Blissful Health

by

Dr.VIJAYALAKSHMI ALURI

FREE VALUABLE POSTS FOR YOU

"I cannot teach anybody anything, I can only make them THINK." - Socrates

Assure you to forward valuable posts!

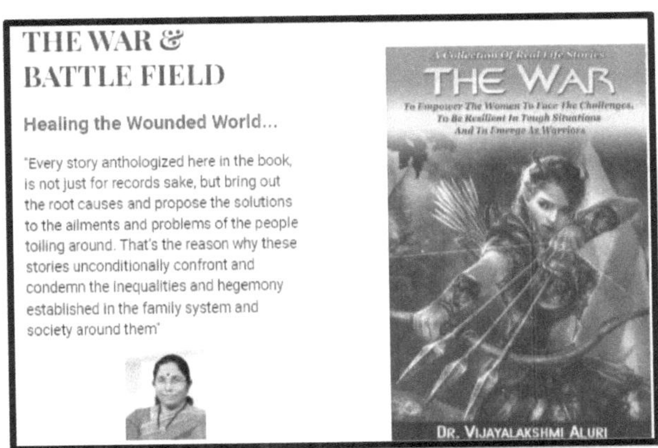

Scan the QR code below to subscribe!

DEDICATION

To

All The Women In General

&

All The Mothers in Particular

WHY YOU SHOULD READ THIS BOOK?

"Celebrate Your Pregnancy" is not just a book; it's your companion, confidant, and guide on the path to motherhood. Whether you're a first-time mom or adding to your family, this book empowers you with knowledge, celebrates the beauty of pregnancy, and provides practical advice for a healthy and joyful experience. From conception to childbirth, this book is your go-to resource for embracing every moment and Celebrating the miracle of life within.

It's time to revel in the magic – you deserve to celebrate your pregnancy!

Having a baby is one of the most exciting things that can happen to you. But you might be feeling nervous as well. If it's your first baby, it's hard to know what to expect.

Your friends, relatives, colleagues, neighbours and your mom or sisters, all of them might be giving you advice on your journey of safe pregnancy.

Moreover there is abundant information on the internet as well as in magazines and books. At times it can be confusing making it difficult to know what to follow and what to avoid.

The guidance and guidelines do change over time with the advancements in research and new tools of care.

So it is important to get up-to-date, practical knowledge and trusted advice to empower you to make the right decisions and follow healthy choices. This book addresses that most crucial need in your life.

Why "Celebrate Your Pregnancy" Is a Must-Read?

"Celebrate Your Pregnancy" is more than just a book; it's an empowering companion that resonates with the whispers of hope within every expectant parent.

This comprehensive guide not only weaves a touching narrative of a couple's journey but also provides invaluable insights into the common discomforts, emotional shifts, and hormonal changes that define the pregnancy experience.

Whether you're on your own journey to parenthood or seeking to empathize with the challenges faced by others, **"Whispers of Hope"** and **"Celebrate Your Pregnancy"** together form a captivating duet that celebrates the strength, resilience, and sheer joy that comes with bringing new life into the world. Immerse yourself in the enchanting tale, find solace in shared experiences, and celebrate the whispers of hope that accompany the miracle of pregnancy.

PREFACE

The incredible journey of pregnancy

The Miracle Begins

The Marvel of Conception

The journey of pregnancy begins with conception, the miraculous fusion of an egg and sperm. Once fertilized, the fertilized egg, known as a **zygote**, embarks on an incredible expedition. It travels through the fallopian tube, multiplying rapidly as it heads toward the uterus. This journey, although minuscule in scale, sets the stage for the extraordinary transformations to come.

The Miracle Unfolds: Conception and the Beginning of Life

Conception marks the inception of an extraordinary journey—a microscopic union that sets in motion the creation of life. It begins with the meeting of two singular cells—the egg and the sperm—in a breath-taking act of biological synchronicity.

In the depths of the female reproductive system, a mature egg, released from the ovary during ovulation, awaits its destined encounter. Simultaneously, millions of tiny, resilient sperm cells embark on a mission, navigating through the intricate labyrinth of the female reproductive tract.

Upon reaching the fallopian tube, where the egg gracefully lingers, the sperm begin their arduous yet awe-inspiring race towards a singular goal: **fertilization.** Among the multitude of contenders, only one fortunate sperm cell will succeed in penetrating the egg's protective barrier—a process known as **fertilization.**

This remarkable event initiates a sequence of transformations that are nothing short of miraculous. The union of genetic material from both the egg and the sperm forms a **zygote**—a single cell imbued with the **complete blueprint of a new life**. This tiny but burgeoning entity holds the potential for an entire human being, encapsulating the intricate code that will define its **physical attributes, personality traits,** and more.

As the zygote begins its clandestine journey down the fallopian tube, it rapidly divides and multiplies—a testament to the unfathomable complexities of cellular growth. With each division, the cluster of cells evolves, forming a **blastocyst** that eventually implants itself into the uterine lining, signalling the inception of pregnancy.

The profound intricacies of conception are beyond mere chance or randomness—they underscore the marvel of biology, the synchronicity of life, and the beginning of an incomparable journey. From this initial union springs forth the wonder of human existence, heralding the onset of the profound transformation that is pregnancy.

Conception, with its astonishing orchestration of cellular events, marks the **genesis of a new chapter—a chapter** brimming with promise, hope, and the boundless potential of life itself. It is the genesis of a miraculous journey, one that will unfold with each passing moment, guiding the formation and growth of a new being—a journey that begins with the miraculous embrace of a single cell.

DESCRIPTION

Celebrate Your Pregnancy: A Holistic Guide to
Embracing the Journey

Are you expecting a bundle of joy and eager to revel in the miracle of pregnancy? Look no further – "Celebrate Your Pregnancy" is the comprehensive guide you've been waiting for. This book is your trusted companion throughout the transformative journey of pregnancy, offering insights, advice, and celebrations for each step along the way

Learning the basics of pregnancy:

Uncover the mysteries of conception as we delve into the fundamentals of starting this incredible journey. From understanding ovulation to demystifying fertility, this chapter sets the stage for the adventure that lies ahead

Preconceptional counseling

Prepare your mind and body for the journey ahead with expert advice on preconceptional counseling. Learn about lifestyle adjustments, health assessments, and key considerations to optimize your chances of a healthy pregnancy.

Whispers of Hope: Celebrate Your Pregnancy Journey:

Embark on an emotionally charged and uplifting journey with "Whispers of Hope," a heartwarming tale of a couple's resilient desire to welcome a child into their lives after a prolonged wait. This enchanting story unfolds like a gentle melody, resonating with the universal themes of love, patience, and the unwavering hope that accompanies the journey to parenthood.

Physical, changes in the mother in different stages of pregnancy

Explore the intricate tapestry of changes your body undergoes during pregnancy. From the emotional rollercoaster to the physical adaptations, gain a deeper understanding of the incredible transformation taking place within you.

Growth and development of fetus week by week

Witness the miracle of life unfold as we guide you through the fetal development journey, week by week. From the first fluttering movements to the development of vital organs, every milestone is a celebration.

Emotional changes during pregnancy

Experience the ebb and flow of emotions that characterize the expectant mother's journey. From the joyous highs to the moments of vulnerability, "Whispers of Hope" beautifully captures the emotional nuances of pregnancy, providing a poignant portrayal of the emotional tapestry that accompanies the creation of life.

Hormonal changes during pregnancy:

Peer into the intricacies of the hormonal symphony that orchestrates the miracle of life within. **"Whispers of Hope"** explores the physiological changes that occur during pregnancy, offering readers a deeper understanding of the incredible transformations happening within the expectant mother's body

Antenatal care:

Delve into the importance of antenatal care as we guide you through the various aspects of healthcare during pregnancy.

From regular check-ups to specialized consultations, prioritize your well-being and that of your baby.

Marvel at the astounding adaptability of the female body during pregnancy. Uncover the secrets of the uterus, hormonal fluctuations, and the remarkable adjustments that make your body the perfect vessel for new life

Routine tests during pregnancy

Navigate the world of routine tests with confidence. Understand the importance of prenatal screenings, diagnostic tests, and monitoring your baby's health, ensuring a smooth and informed pregnancy experience.

Overview of your Pregnancy care: Step into the shoes of the protagonists as they navigate the labyrinth of emotions, setbacks, and triumphs on the path to parenthood.

From the initial spark of hope to the exhilarating moments of discovery, witness the couple's transformative journey with every turn of the page.

Common discomforts during pregnancy

As the story unfolds, delve into the reality of pregnancy as the expectant mother experiences the common discomforts that come with carrying new life. "Whispers of Hope" sheds light on the challenges, offering a comforting and informative perspective on how to navigate them with grace.

Self -care during pregnancy

Prioritize your well-being with insights into nutrition, exercise, and self-care tailored for the expectant mother. Discover the art of nourishing your body, staying active safely, and embracing self-love during this joyous journey.

TABLE OF CONTENTS

NUTRITION AND LIFE STYLE DURING PREGNANCY.................147

CHAPTER: 1

LEARNING THE BASICS OF CONCEPTION

Desires to get pregnant?

So, you and your partner are ready to have a child.

Congratulations!

You probably know what must happen next: **Sperm must meet egg.** To become pregnant, the couple should have sex around the time of ovulation, the time when an ovary releases an egg .

Know your menstrual cycle

To get pregnant, you need to know when ovulation happens. You are most fertile around the time an egg is released, and this is when you should plan to have sex.

Track your periods on a calendar: The easiest and least expensive way to figure out when you are ovulating is to tracking your periods. **Ovulation typically happens about 14 days before your period starts.** This is rather consistent from person to person, no matter how long your menstrual cycle is.

Do you want to understand how the days of the menstrual cycle are counted?

A menstrual cycle lasts from the first day of your period to the first day of your next period. So if your period starts on July 1, that's day 1.

From here, determining your most fertile days takes just a little bit of mathematics. If your cycle is normally **21 days long**, then you likely **ovulate around day 7 (21 minus 14 equals 7)**. If your cycle is on the longer side, say **35 days**, you ovulate around day 21. If your cycle ranges between 26 and 28 days long, then ovulation happens between days **12 and 14** in any given cycle.

Monitoring cervical mucus: It also helps to notice changes in your body. Of all the methods to self-detect ovulation, **monitoring cervical mucus** tends to be the most reliable.

Cervical mucus is a type of vaginal discharge: The mucus comes from your cervix and exits through the vagina. This mucus changes throughout the month and **peaks 1 to 2 days before ovulation.** At this point in your cycle, you may notice **a clear vaginal discharge that feels thin and stretchy.**

There is no fool proof way to calculate your fertile days. But knowing the pattern of your menstrual cycle and changes in your cervical mucus can give you a pretty good sense of when to have sex.

When to have sex?

There is no ideal moment when the couple must have sex. **The window of fertility** is about **6 days** each cycle. This is because **sperm can live in a woman's body for as long as 5 days**, while an **egg can survive for about 12 to 24 hours after ovulation**. So **you can have sex up to 5 days before ovulation or 1 day after** and **still get pregnant**.

For the best chance of getting pregnant, research suggests that **you should have sex every day or every other day during this 6-day window.**

Avoid investing in extra tools.

Today there are innumerable smartphone apps, devices, and other tools on the market designed to help you get pregnant as soon as possible. These range from free period tracking apps to ovulation predictor kits you can buy at the drugstore for about $20. Some more sophisticated devices can cost hundreds of dollars.

These tools can certainly help you track and notice trends in your menstrual cycle. They are also **useful if you and your partner only have sex once or twice a month,** in which case you really need to pinpoint the best time to get pregnant.

On the other hand, fertility trackers and ovulation predictors can create a sense of urgency around getting pregnant and make you tensed up. Many people find the information overwhelming and become fixated on doing everything **"just right."**

Moreover, these tools don't work for everybody, and the results are not always accurate. For example, if you have highly irregular periods, trying to predict ovulation at home is not going to be worth your time or money.

Instead seek advice from an ob-gyn. Highly irregular periods may be a sign you are not ovulating, and you may need medications that can help make you ovulate.

There's also concern about period tracking apps and the privacy of your health data. If you're thinking about using an app, first review how it would store and share your data.

Take Note: These tools can be nice to have but are unnecessary for most couples. The costs may outweigh the benefits, especially if they create anxiety.

Use the technology only as much as it suits you.

When to talk with your ob-gyn?

You can't expect to get pregnant right away. More than half of healthy couples get pregnant within the first 6 months of trying. This can be difficult to accept when you want to have a child very soon.

But, if you're under 35 and have been trying for an entire year without success, contact your ob-gyn.

The problem is most likely to be that you're not having sex often enough or at the right time. If you are 35 to 39, you should seek help after 6 months of trying. And if you're 40 or older, better to seek help even sooner.

Having a Baby After Age 35: How Aging Affects Fertility and Pregnancy?

After age 35, there's a **higher risk of pregnancy-related complications that might lead to a C-section delivery**. The risk of chromosomal conditions is higher. Babies born to older mothers have a higher risk of certain chromosomal conditions, such as **Down syndrome.** The risk of pregnancy **loss** is higher.

If you have a history of **endometriosis, polycystic ovary syndrome (PCOS), or prior pelvic surgery,** it is harder to get pregnant. In these cases, it's a good idea to see a fertility specialist early on.

For most couples, the prospect of getting pregnant can feel both anxious and exciting.

Hopefully, you will succeed within a few months. If you don't, there are ways to figure out the problem and improve your chances.

Consult your ob-gyn or a reproductive endocrinologist, they will be able to help and guide you through this journey.

CHAPTER: 2

COMPREHENSIVE PRECONCEPTION COUNSELLING

Preconception counselling and **screening** are essential components of reproductive healthcare aimed at optimizing maternal and foetal health before conception.

This proactive approach involves **comprehensive discussions, evaluations**, and **interventions** to identify and address potential risks and promote a healthy pregnancy.

Preconception counselling is also a **comprehensive, individualized evaluation** and **planning process** that helps women prepare for pregnancy and optimize their health prior to conception.

During preconception counselling, a healthcare provider will assess the woman's current health status, identify any potential health risks, and make recommendations for optimizing health before conception.

Preconception counselling includes:

I. MEDICAL HISTORY ASSESSMENT

Medical history assessment during preconception counselling involves a thorough exploration of a **woman's health history**, aiming to identify any **existing conditions, past pregnancies, surgeries, medications,** and **family medical background** that might impact her or her potential baby's health. Here's a detailed breakdown

Elements of medical history assessment:

A. Chronic health conditions

How chronic health conditions such as **diabetes, hypertension, thyroid disorders, epilepsy** and **autoimmune diseases** might affect pregnancy would be discussed.

B. Reproductive Health

History of **menstrual irregularities, polycystic ovary syndrome (PCOS), endometriosis**, or any previous reproductive health issues

C. Previous pregnancies

Details about previous pregnancies, including complications, deliveries, miscarriages, or any history of preterm labour would be analysed.

D. Gynaecological history

Information about **pelvic inflammatory disease (PID), sexually transmitted infections** and **gynaecological surgeries** would be noted.

E. Medication and supplements review

Comprehensive discussion about current medications, including prescription drugs, over-the-counter medications, supplements, vitamins, and herbal remedies. Their safety during pregnancy would be evaluated.

F. Allergies and reactions

Identification of any known allergies or adverse reactions to medications, foods, environmental elements, or substances that might pose risks during pregnancy would be done.

G. Family medical history

Investigation into family medical history, including **genetic conditions, congenital anomalies**, **inherited disorders,** and any history of pregnancy-related complications (e.g., **preeclampsia, gestational diabetes**)

H. Lifestyle factors

Lifestyle elements such as smoking, alcohol consumption, drug use, caffeine intake, diet, exercise habits, and exposure to environmental toxins or hazards would be assessed.

I. Psychosocial History

Evaluation of mental health history, including stress levels, anxiety, depression, and any previous experiences of postpartum depression or other mental health conditions

Significance of Medical History Assessment

1. Risk identification

The potential risk factors that might affect fertility, pregnancy, or the health of the unborn child would be recognised mostly.

2. Risk mitigations

Allows healthcare providers to formulate personalized plans to manage existing conditions, adjust medications if necessary, and mitigate potential risks before conception.

3. Optimization of pregnancy outcome

Understanding the medical history assists in creating a **tailored preconception care plan,** leading to a healthier pregnancy and better outcomes for both mother and child.

A comprehensive medical history assessment is integral in tailoring preconception care, ensuring a smooth and healthy journey through pregnancy and childbirth.

II. LIFE STYLE EVALUATION

Discussions around lifestyle factors such as **smoking, alcohol consumption, drug use, diet, exercise** and **environmental exposures** are crucial. Recommendations for necessary lifestyle changes are made to optimize health.

Evaluating lifestyle factors is crucial as it helps identify areas for improvement and empowers women to make informed choices that optimize their health and increase the likelihood of a healthy pregnancy.

Detailed overview of lifestyle evaluation in preconception counselling:

Elements of Lifestyle Evaluation

1. Smoking, alcohol and substance use

Smoking

Encourage to avoid **smoking** by making the woman aware of the adverse effects of smoking on fertility, pregnancy complications, and foetal development.

Alcohol and drug use

Discussing the risks associated with alcohol consumption and illicit drug use during conception and pregnancy

2. Dietary habits

Nutritional assessment

Reviewing dietary habits to ensure adequate intake of essential nutrients like folic acid, iron, calcium, and vitamins is crucial for foetal development.

3. Weight management

Addressing issues related to being underweight or overweight, and providing guidance on healthy weight management.

4. Physical activity

Exercise guidelines

Providing recommendations for safe and appropriate physical activity levels during preconception and pregnancy to maintain overall health.

5. Stress and Mental Health

Stress management

Discussing stress management techniques and coping strategies as chronic stress can impact fertility and pregnancy outcomes.

Mental health support

Identifying any history of anxiety, depression, or other mental health concerns and providing support or referrals as needed.

6. Occupational and environmental exposures

Workplace hazards

Identifying any history of anxiety, depression, or other mental health concerns and providing support or referrals as needed.

Environmental toxins

Discussing potential exposure to environmental toxins or pollutants that could affect fertility or pregnancy.

7. Recreational advises

Discussing travel plans and potential risks associated with certain activities or destinations during preconception and pregnancy.

Importance of lifestyle evaluation

Optimizing Fertility

Addressing lifestyle factors that may negatively impact fertility, aiming to enhance the chances of conception.

Reducing Pregnancy Risks

Modifying habits to reduce the risk of complications during pregnancy, such as preterm birth, low birth weight, or birth defects.

Promoting foetal development

Ensuring an optimal environment for the developing foetus by adopting healthy lifestyle choices before conception.

Personalised guidance and support

Healthcare providers offer personalized advice, guidance, and support based on the individual's lifestyle choices and needs. Encouraging healthy habits and addressing potential risks through lifestyle evaluation plays a significant role in preparing for a successful and healthy pregnancy

III. NUTRITIONAL GUIDANCE

During the preconception stage, focusing on nutrition is crucial as it can impact both partners' fertility and the health of the future baby.

Key points for nutritional guidance during preconception phase:

Healthy diet:

Encourage a well-balanced diet rich in fruits, vegetables, whole grains, lean proteins, and healthy fats. A diverse diet provides essential vitamins and minerals necessary for reproductive health.

Maintain healthy diet:

Both underweight and overweight can affect fertility. Aim for a healthy weight range, as extremes can impact hormone levels and reproductive functions.

Folate and Folic acid:

Adequate intake of folic acid is vital to reduce the risk of neural tube defects in the baby. It's recommended to take a folic acid supplement (400 to 800 micrograms per day) before conception and during the first trimester.

Omege-3 fatty acids:

Found in fatty fish, flaxseeds, and walnuts, omega-3 fatty acids are beneficial for reproductive health. They help regulate hormones and promote healthy egg and sperm development.

Limit processed foods and Trans fats:

Diets high in processed foods and Trans fats can impact fertility negatively. Opt for whole, unprocessed foods and healthier fat sources

Stay hydrated:

Drinking enough water is essential for overall health and can support reproductive functions.

Supplements:

Alongside folic acid, consider prenatal vitamins containing iron, calcium, vitamin D, and other essential nutrients. Consult a healthcare provider for personalized   advice.

Adequate intake of essential nutrients like **folic acid, iron, calcium**, and **other vitamins** is emphasized. Recommendations might include **starting prenatal vitamins before conception.**

Remember, individual nutritional needs vary, and it's essential to consult with a healthcare provider or a registered dietician for personalized guidance and recommendations based on specific health conditions, lifestyle, and dietary preferences

Limit caffeine and alcohol:

High caffeine intake has been linked to decreased fertility, and excessive alcohol consumption can negatively impact conception and foetal development.

IV. CHRONIC DISEASES MANAGEMENT

Women with chronic conditions like **diabetes, hypertension, thyroid disorders**, or **epilepsy** need specialized care to stabilize these conditions before conception to reduce risks during pregnancy.

Preconception counselling for individuals with chronic diseases involves specialized guidance and planning to manage health conditions before attempting pregnancy.

1. Diabetes

Blood sugar control: Achieving and maintaining optimal blood sugar levels before conception lowers the risk of birth defects. Healthcare providers may adjust medication, diet, and exercise routines.

Folic acid supplementation: Essential for women with diabetes as it helps prevent neural tube defects.

Regular monitoring: Consistent blood sugar monitoring is crucial, as fluctuations can occur more frequently during pregnancy

2. Hypertension(High blood pressure)

Medication review: Some blood pressure medications are not safe during pregnancy. Healthcare providers might switch to safer alternatives. Angiotensin-converting enzyme inhibitors (**ACE inhibitors**), Angiotensin receptor blockers (**ARBs**) and **Renin inhibitors** are not safe to use in pregnancy.

Healthy life style: Emphasize a **heart-healthy diet** low in sodium, regular exercise, and stress management techniques.

3. Thyroid disorders

Thyroid hormone regulation: Ensure thyroid hormone levels are stable and within the normal range before conception. Medication adjustments might be necessary.

Monitoring: Regular thyroid function tests to maintain optimal levels throughout pregnancy.

4. Autoimmune diseases (e.g. Lupus, Rheumatoid arthritis):

Medication adjustment: Some medications might need to be adjusted or changed to safer alternatives before conception.

Consult specialists: Coordination with rheumatologists or specialists to optimize treatment plans.

5. Epilepsy

Medication review: Certain anti-seizure medications may pose risks during pregnancy. Healthcare providers may adjust doses or switch to safer alternatives.

Folic acid supplementation: Important to reduce the risk of birth defects

6. Obesity

Weight management: Achieving a healthy weight before conception reduces the risk of complications during pregnancy. Healthcare providers can offer guidance on diet and exercise plans.

7. Celiac diseases and digestive disorders: Ensuring proper absorption of nutrients through diet or supplements. Proper management can prevent deficiencies that might affect pregnancy

8. Mental health conditions

Medication review Evaluate the safety of psychiatric medications during pregnancy. Some might need adjustment or change.

Psychological support: Preconception counselling to address mental health concerns and stress management techniques.

Preconception counselling includes screening for various infectious diseases to ensure a healthy pregnancy and reduce the risk of transmission to the baby. Screening for infectious diseases before conception helps identify and manage potential risks.

Key infectious diseases often screened for during preconception counselling:

A. Rubella (German measles): Rubella can cause severe birth defects if contracted during pregnancy. Women are typically screened for immunity through a blood test. If a woman is not immune, vaccination is recommended before conception.

B. Varicella (Chicken pox): Similar to rubella, contracting chickenpox during pregnancy can lead to birth defects. Testing for immunity is advisable, and vaccination is suggested for non-immune individuals before conception.

C. HIV (Human immunodeficiency virus): Testing for HIV is crucial for both partners. If one partner is HIV-positive, steps can be taken to minimize the risk of transmission to the other partner and reduce the risk of transmitting the virus to the baby.

D. Hepatitis B and C: Screening for hepatitis B and C helps in identifying carriers and preventing transmission to the baby. Vaccination and medical management can be initiated if necessary.

E. Toxoplasmosis: Toxoplasmosis can be a sexually transmitted infection with serious clinical consequences. Not all routes of infection are created equal.

This infection can cause severe problems for the foetus if contracted during pregnancy. In the neonate, manifestations of **congenital toxoplasmosis** might include **hydrocephalus, microcephaly, intracranial calcifications, retinochoroiditis, strabismus, blindness, epilepsy, psychomotor** and **mental retardation, petechiae due to thrombocytopenia,** and **anaemia.**

F. Cytomegalovirus (CMV): CMV can cause birth defects if a woman contracts it for the first time during pregnancy. While routine screening is less common, understanding potential risks and preventive measures can be part of counselling.

If a pregnant woman is infected with CMV, she can pass it to her developing baby. This is called congenital CMV, and it can cause birth defects and other health problems.

Infants born with signs of congenital CMV disease at birth will have long-term health problems, such as: **Hearing loss**, Vision **loss, Intellectual disability**.

Preconception infectious disease screening aims to identify and manage infections that could affect pregnancy outcomes. Depending on the individual's medical history, risk factors, and potential exposures, healthcare providers may recommend additional tests or vaccinations.

Screening may be recommended, especially for women who work with or have frequent exposure to cats or raw meat.

If infections are identified, appropriate treatments or preventive measures are often initiated before attempting conception to promote a healthy pregnancy and protect the well-being of both the parent and the baby

VI. GENETIC COUNSELLING AND TESTING

Assessing the need for genetic testing based on family history to identify potential genetic disorders or carrier status that could affect the offspring.

Genetic counselling and testing in preconception care involve evaluating the risk of passing on genetic disorders to offspring.

A. Family history assessment: Genetic counsellors collect detailed family health histories to identify any patterns of inherited conditions or genetic disorders.

B. Risk assessment: Based on family history and ethnic background, counsellors assess the risk of passing on genetic conditions. This assessment helps in determining the need for specific genetic tests.

C. Carrier screening: Genetic testing may be recommended to identify whether either partner carries genetic mutations for conditions like **cystic fibrosis, sickle cell disease, Tay-Sachs disease, thalassemia, etc**. Carrier status does not mean the person has the condition but indicates the **potential to pass it on to their child**.

D. Ethnicity specific Testing: Certain genetic disorders are more prevalent in specific ethnic groups. For instance, Tay-Sachs disease is more common among individuals of Ashkenazi Jewish descent. Therefore, targeted tests may be suggested based on ethnic backgrounds.

E. Genetic counselling: After assessing the results, genetic counsellors provide detailed information about the condition, its inheritance patterns, and the potential implications for future offspring. They discuss available options, such as **prenatal testing, preimplantation genetic diagnosis (PGD), or adoption**, depending on the specific genetic risk identified.

F. Prenatal testing options: Couples identified as high-risk based on carrier screening or family history may opt for prenatal testing during pregnancy to further assess the foetus for specific genetic conditions.

G. Pre-implantation Genetic testing: In vitro fertilization **(IVF)** combined with preimplantation genetic testing allows the selection of embryos free from specific genetic conditions before implantation.

H. Decision making support: Genetic counsellors offer support in decision-making, considering the emotional, ethical, and practical aspects associated with potential genetic risks.

Overall, genetic counselling and testing in preconception care **aim to inform couples about the potential genetic risks** they might face and **offer options** to make informed decisions about family planning.

It empowers individuals to understand their genetic makeup, assess risks, and take proactive steps to minimize the chances of passing on genetic disorders to their children.

VII. REPRODUCTIVE PLANNING

Reproductive planning within preconception counselling involves discussions and strategies to help individuals or couples achieve their family planning goals.

A. Timing of conception: Discussing the optimal timing for conception based on individual circumstances, such as age, health, and life goals. This includes considerations about when to start trying to conceive and potential factors that may affect fertility.

B. Fertility Awareness: Educating individuals about the **menstrual cycle, ovulation,** and **fertile windows**

can assist in maximizing the chances of conception. This may involve methods like **tracking menstrual cycles, basal body temperature charting,** and **ovulation predictor kits**.

C. Health optimization: Emphasizing the importance of optimizing health before conception. This includes maintaining a **healthy weight, managing chronic conditions, adopting a balanced diet,** and **ensuring regular exercise** and **adequate sleep.**

D. Folic acid supplementation: Recommending folic acid supplementation (**400 to 800 micrograms per day**) before conception to reduce the risk of neural tube defects in the baby.

E. Environmental and lifestyle factors: Discussing the impact of lifestyle choices, such as smoking, alcohol consumption, and exposure to environmental toxins, on fertility and the health of the future baby. Advising on necessary lifestyle changes to create a conducive environment for conception.

F. Medical history review: Evaluating the medical history of both partners to identify any potential risks or concerns that may affect fertility or pregnancy. Addressing underlying health issues before conception can optimize outcomes.

G. Reproductive health screening: Conducting tests to assess reproductive health, such as checking for **sexually**

transmitted infections (STIs), hormone levels, and other factors that might affect fertility.

H. Contraception discussion: If transitioning from contraception to planning for pregnancy, discussing the different methods, their cessation timeline, and potential considerations for fertility return after discontinuation.

I. Sexual health and intimacy: Encouraging open discussions about sexual health, intimacy, and any concerns or questions related to sexual activity around conception.

J. Counselling on emotional and psychological readiness: Preparing mentally and emotionally for parenthood, addressing any concerns, and providing support in navigating the emotional aspects of family planning.

Reproductive planning in preconception counselling aims to empower individuals or couples with the knowledge, resources, and support needed to make informed decisions about starting a family while optimizing their chances of a healthy conception, pregnancy, and childbirth.

Discussions about fertility awareness, contraception discontinuation, and timing of conception based on menstrual cycles are vital.

VIII. SCREENING AND INVESTIGATIONS

Blood tests:

- Complete blood count (CBC), blood type and Rh factor, screening for anaemia checking immunity to certain infections, and thyroid function tests.

- Pap smear and pelvic examination

- To screen for cervical cancer and assess pelvic health.

Immunizations:

Ensuring up-to-date vaccinations, especially for rubella, varicella, and influenza.

Some vaccines are not recommended during pregnancy, such as:

- Human papillomavirus (HPV) vaccine.

- Measles, mumps, and rubella (MMR) vaccine.

- Live influenza vaccine (nasal flu vaccine)

- Varicella (chicken pox) vaccine.

- Certain travel vaccines: yellow fever, typhoid fever, and Japanese encephalitis

Urine tests:

Screening for urinary tract infections and other urinary abnormalities.

Genetic screening

Based on family history, ethnic background, or previous pregnancies, to do tests to assess the risk of genetic conditions in the offspring.

Additional considerations

Counselling on medications:

Review and adjustment of any medications that might pose risks during pregnancy

Mental Health screening:

Assessing mental health conditions and providing necessary support.

BMI and weight evaluation

Discussing weight management and its impact on fertility and pregnancy.

Preconception care is personalized based on individual health needs and helps ensure a healthier pregnancy and a better start for the baby. Consulting a healthcare provider for preconception counselling is highly recommended for women planning to conceive. In all cases, preconception counselling involves close collaboration between healthcare providers, including specialists, to ensure a comprehensive evaluation of the individual's health status and tailored management plans. Regular check-ups, lifestyle modifications, and medication adjustments are crucial elements to optimize health before attempting pregnancy, reducing risks to both the parent and the baby.

CHAPTER: 3

WHISPERS OF HOPE: A JOURNEY TO PARENTHOOD

Once upon a time, nestled in the heart of a small town, there lived a couple, Sarah and Jack, who dreamt of a life filled with the pitter-patter of little feet and the joy of parenthood. They were high school sweethearts, bound by a love that grew stronger with each passing day. Yet, as they strolled through the colourful streets, hand in hand, a silent longing echoed within their hearts.

Their desire for a child was not just a fleeting wish but a fervent dream they held close. They yearned for the laughter that would fill their home, for tiny hands that would grasp theirs, and for the miracle of life growing within Sarah's womb.

Months turned into years, and their hope wavered as they faced the silent whispers of disappointment month after month. Each negative test felt like a crushing blow, leaving behind fragments of shattered dreams. The laughter that once echoed through their home seemed to fade, replaced by a palpable ache that settled between them.

But their love remained resilient, a beacon of hope in the face of adversity. They decided to seek guidance, to explore the possibilities, and to unravel the mysteries that thwarted their journey toward parenthood. With a glimmer of hope, they embarked on a new chapter in their lives - preconception counselling.

Dr Evelyn, a gentle and empathetic obstetrician, welcomed them into her cozy clinic adorned with hues of tranquillity. Her warm smile instantly put Sarah and Jack at ease as they settled into comfortable chairs, surrounded by walls adorned with stories of hope and triumph.

Dr. Evelyn listened intently as they poured their hearts out, sharing their aspirations, fears, and the rollercoaster of emotions that defined their quest for a child. She offered them solace, assuring them that their journey was not one they had to traverse alone.

"Embarking on the journey of parenthood is an incredible adventure," She began, her voice a soothing melody. "But it's not always a straightforward path. Sometimes, it takes a little guidance, a touch of science, and a lot of faith."

Under her guidance, Sarah and Jack delved into the depths of preconception counselling. They learned about the intricate dance of hormones, the significance of a healthy lifestyle, and the importance of patience and understanding. Dr.Evelyn became their guiding light, leading them through a labyrinth of medical jargon with compassion and clarity. They discovered the beauty of synchronization between mind, body, and soul. Meditation sessions brought a sense of serenity to their hectic lives, and yoga became a shared ritual that united their spirits. Together, they embraced a nutritious diet, savoring each meal as a step towards nurturing the life they yearned to create.

As they delved deeper into their journey, Sarah and Jack found solace in each other's embrace. They discovered a newfound strength in their unity, transforming challenges into opportunities for growth. They immersed themselves in the beauty of nature, finding solace in the rustling leaves and the tranquillity of starlit skies, reminding them of the vastness of possibilities.

Months passed, marked by the rhythm of their newfound routine, their hearts resilient against the tides of uncertainty. And then, one serene evening, as the sun painted the sky in hues of orange and gold, Sarah felt a stirring within her—a whisper from within that felt like a miracle unfolding.

A visit to Dr Evelyn confirmed their greatest joy. They sat hand in hand, tears of elation glistening in their eyes, as they heard the unmistakable sound of a tiny heartbeat echoing through the room—a symphony of hope, resilience, and unwavering love.

Their journey had been a tapestry woven with threads of courage, patience, and unyielding faith. As they walked out of the clinic, embraced by the warmth of the setting sun, Sarah rested her head on Jack's shoulder, their hearts brimming with gratitude for the miracle that awaited them—a new chapter, a precious life, and the beginning of their greatest adventure yet.

CHAPTER: 4

GETTING PREGNANT: EMBARKING ON LIFE'S JOURNEY

Exploring Ovulation, Fertilization, Implantation, and the Dawn of Early Pregnancy

OVULATION

Ovulation occurs each month when an egg (ovum) is released from one of the ovaries.

Ovulation or release of egg from the ovary, occurs about **14 days before** the next menstrual period and the ovum is swept into the funnel-shaped end of one of the fallopian tubes.

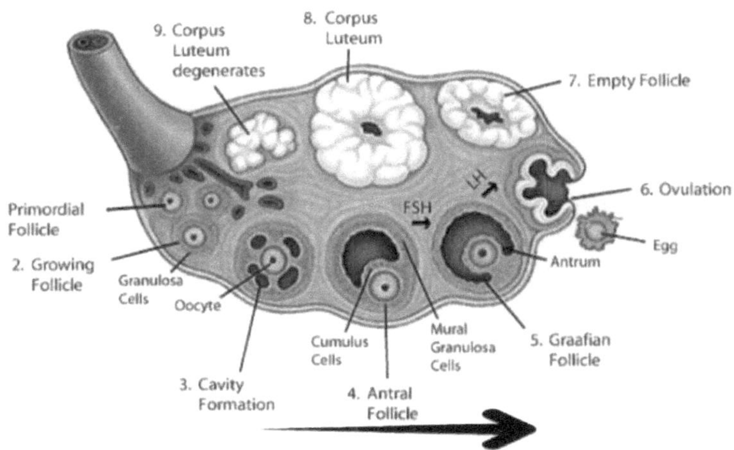

FERTILISATION

During sex, sperm are ejaculated from a man's penis into a woman's vagina. In one ejaculation there may be more than 300 million sperm. Most of the sperm leak out of the vagina but some begin to swim up through the cervix. When a woman is ovulating, the mucus in the cervix is thinner than usual to let sperm pass through more easily. Sperm swim into the uterus and into the fallopian tubes. If a female and male have **sex within 12-24 hours** of the **female's ovulation**, spermatozoa that are deposited in the vagina swim up through the cervix and uterus, enter the fallopian tubes and one of the spermatozoa penetrates the egg, forming the **zygote**.

Cilia, Tiny hair like structures lining the fallopian tube propel the fertilized egg (**zygote**) through the tube towards the uterus. The cells of the zygote divide repeatedly as the zygote moves down the fallopian tube. The zygote enters the uterus in 3 to 5 days.

If the egg is not fertilised, the egg degenerates and will pass out of the body during the woman's monthly period along with the lining of the uterus, which is also shed.

DEVELOPMENT OF THE BLASTOCYST & IMPLANTATION

- During the week after fertilisation, the fertilised egg moves slowly down the fallopian tube and into the uterus.

- About a week after the fertilization, the fertilized egg (**zygote**) has become a multicelled **blastocyst.**

- During pregnancy, your hormone levels change. As soon as you have conceived, the amount of oestrogen and progesterone in your blood increases. This causes the uterus lining to build up, the blood supply to your uterus and breasts to increase and the muscles of your uterus to relax to make room for the growing baby.

- Oestrogen and Progesterone cause the endometrium to become thick and rich with blood making it spongy, so that the blastocyst burrows itself into this **specially thickened** endometrium and absorb nutrients from it. This process is called **Implantation** which is completed by **day 9 or 10**.

- The wall of the **blastocyst** is one cell thick except in one area, where it is three to four cells thick. The inner cells in the thickened area develop into the embryo, and the outer cells burrow into the wall of the uterus and develop into the placenta.

- The placenta produces **human chorionic gonadotropin,** that help maintain the pregnancy and prevents the ovaries from releasing eggs and stimulates the ovaries to produce oestrogen and progesterone continuously.

- Oxygen and nutrition from the mother is supplied to the foetus and waste materials are carried from the foetus to the mother through the **umbilical cord** which connects the foetus and **placenta.**

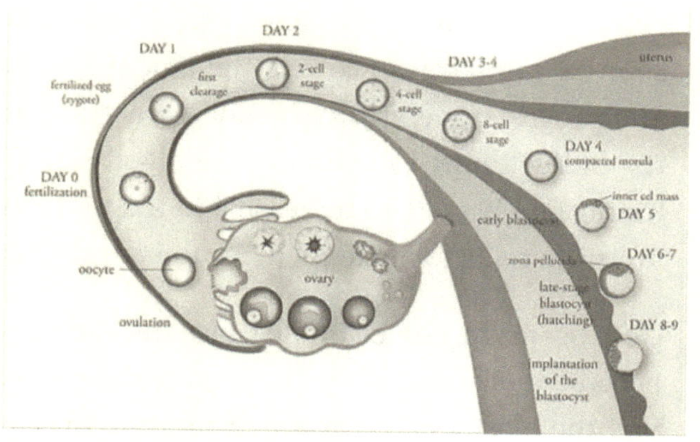

FETAL DEVELOPMENT

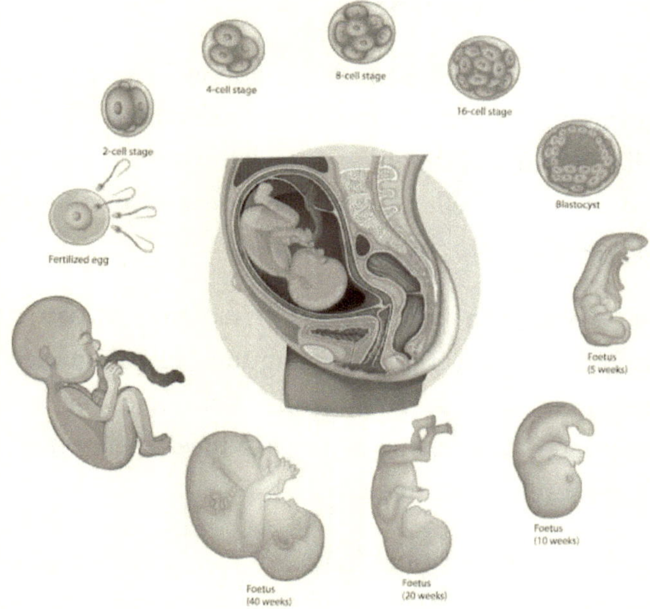

BOY OR GIRL?

Every normal human cell contains 46 chromosomes, except for male sperm and female eggs. These contain 23 chromosomes each. When a sperm fertilises an egg, the 23 chromosomes from the father pair with the 23 from the mother, making 46 in all.

Chromosomes are tiny, thread-like structures which each carry about 2,000 genes. Genes determine a baby's inherited characteristics, **such as hair and eye colour, blood group, height** and **build.**

A fertilised egg contains one sex chromosome from its mother and one from its father. The sex chromosome from the mother's egg is always the same and is known as the X chromosome. The sex chromosome from the father's sperm can be an X or a Y chromosome.

If the egg is fertilised by a sperm containing a X chromosome, the baby will be a girl (XX). If the sperm contains a Y chromosome, the baby will be a boy (XY).

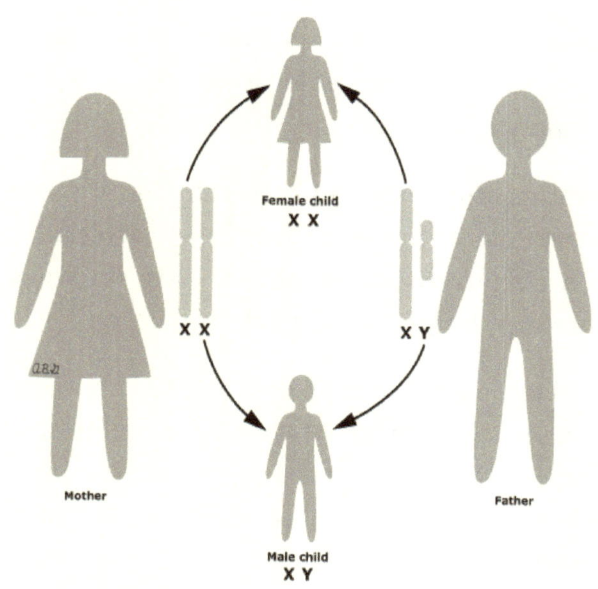

TWINS, TRIPLETS OR MORE

Identical twins occur when one fertilised egg splits into two; each baby will have the same genes – and therefore they will be the same sex and look very alike. Non-identical twins are more common. They are the result of two eggs being fertilised by two sperm at the same time.

The babies may be of the same sex or different sexes, and will probably look no more alike than any other brothers and sisters. A third of all twins will be identical and two-thirds non-identical.

Twins happen in about 1 in every 65 pregnancies. A couple is more likely to have twins if there are twins in the woman's family. Triplets occur naturally in 1 in 10,000 pregnancies and quads are even rarer.

Nowadays, the use of treatments such as in vitro fertilisation (IVF) has made multiple births more common

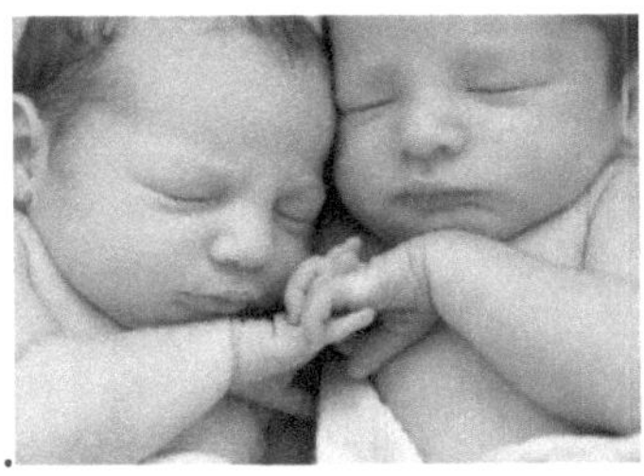

Some facts:

- Even a single intercourse can cause pregnancy

- The sperm determines the sex of the child

- The baby grows in the mother's womb for **280** days, counting from the first day of her last menstrual period.

- Marriage amongst blood relatives (**consanguineous marriage)** increases the chances of abnormal babies.

- Pregnancy should ideally occur **after 19 years** and **before 35 years** of age.

CHAPTER: 5

MIRACLE OF PREGNANCY

Embarking on the Journey: Blossoming new life within you!

The moment you discover that a new life is blossoming within you, the world seems to spin in a different rhythm. It's a symphony of emotions - joy, wonder, maybe a hint of nervousness too, as you step into the exquisite journey of pregnancy.

There's a subtle transformation, not just physically but also within the deepest chambers of your soul. Suddenly, you become a vessel, nurturing a tiny being that will soon call you **"Mom"** or **"Dad."** It's a chapter of life that unfolds with tenderness and anticipation.

FIRST TRIMESTER

Embracing the Secret Symphony: Steering the First Trimester

As the first weeks go by, there's an enchanting secrecy to it all - a shared secret between you and this tiny life that's growing inside. The news might be just between you and your partner, held tight like a precious treasure, waiting for the perfect moment to reveal itself to the world.

The first trimester can be a whirlwind. Amidst the excitement, there might be bouts of morning sickness, a rollercoaster of emotions, and the realization that life is changing in the most beautiful way. There are doctor's appointments, each one marking a milestone - the first ultrasound, the sound of a tiny heartbeat echoing in the room, a visual affirmation of life itself.

Nesting instincts start to kick in. Suddenly, your world revolves around preparing a cozy nest for this new arrival. There's a flurry of baby names whispered in hushed tones, discussions about nursery colours, and the delightful task of choosing tiny clothes that seem impossibly small.

SECOND TRIMESTER

Radiance and Reflection: Voyaging the Second Trimester

The second trimester arrives like a gentle breeze, bringing with it a newfound sense of energy and a radiant glow. The initial worries start to fade, replaced by a sense of confidence and awe at the miracle unfolding within. The baby bump becomes more pronounced, a tangible evidence of the life growing inside.

It's a time when you start feeling those first flutters - subtle movements that remind you of the little one's presence. With every kick, you're reminded of the vitality of this tiny being and the profound connection you share.

Amidst all this, there are moments of reflection. You find yourself marvelling at the sheer miracle of creation, contemplating the enormity of bringing a new life into the world. There's a sense of responsibility, a desire to provide the best possible future for this little soul that's about to grace your world.

Counting Down to Arrival: Embracing the Final Trimester

The third trimester heralds the final stretch of this incredible journey. As the due date draws near, anticipation reaches its peak. There might be moments of discomfort - sleepless nights, aches, and the sheer weight of carrying a precious bundle. But through it all, there's an unwavering excitement and a readiness to embrace what lies ahead.

The **baby shower** becomes a celebration of love and support, surrounded by family and friends who are just as eager to welcome the newest member of the family. Gifts pour in - soft blankets, and toys that will soon fill the nursery with laughter and joy.

As the days pass, you find yourself counting down, eagerly awaiting the first cry, the first touch, and the first gaze into those curious eyes.

The nursery is ready, the bags are packed, and your heart is filled with an indescribable mix of emotions - love, excitement, a touch of nervousness, and a deep sense of gratitude for this extraordinary journey.

Embracing Life's Symphony: Welcoming a New Beginning

And then, the moment arrives - a crescendo in this symphony of life. With a cry that fills the room, a new chapter begins. You hold this precious little being in your arms, feeling a love so overwhelming it takes your breath away. In that moment, you realize that this journey was just the beginning - the beginning of a lifetime of love, joy, and endless wonder as you watch this beautiful soul grow and flourish.

CHAPTER: 6

EMBRACING THE CHANGES

Physical Changes during Pregnancy

Pregnancy is an awe-inspiring journey filled with wonder, anticipation, and transformation. While it's a time of joy and excitement, it's also a period marked by numerous physical changes in a woman's body. Understanding these changes can help expectant mothers travel through this remarkable phase with greater ease and confidence.

How soon can you diagnose pregnancy?

A **missed period** is often the first sign that you may be pregnant, but how do you confirm?

Home urine pregnancy tests are more likely to be accurate when used at least one week after a woman's last period.

A blood test can be done to detect pregnancy sooner than a home pregnancy test.

THE THREE STAGES OF PREGNANCY

A typical pregnancy lasts 40 weeks from the first day of your last menstrual period (LMP) to the birth of the baby. It is divided into three stages, called **trimesters: first trimester, second trimester and third trimester**. The foetus undergoes many changes throughout maturation.

1st Trimester

Conception to about the 12th week of pregnancy marks the first trimester. The second trimester is weeks 13 to 27 weeks, and the third trimester starts about 28 weeks and lasts until birth.

FIRST TRIMESTER: WEEK 1 (CONCEPTION) – WEEK 12

1st trimester pregnancy:

What to expect

The first trimester of pregnancy can be overwhelming. Understand the changes you might experience and how to take care of yourself during this exciting time.

The first trimester of pregnancy is marked by an invisible — yet amazing — transformation. And it happens quickly. Knowing what physical and emotional changes to expect during the first trimester can help you face the months ahead with confidence.

Changes in the first trimester of Pregnancy

As the pregnancy progresses, a woman's body undergoes an array of changes. Hormonal fluctuations play a pivotal role, triggering a cascade of adjustments.

Pregnancy heralds a symphony of transformations within a woman's body, a testament to the remarkable adaptability and resilience of the female form. From the moment conception occurs, a cascade of changes sets in motion, orchestrated by the intricate actions of hormones and physiological adaptations.

While your first sign of pregnancy might have been a missed period, you can expect several other physical changes in the coming weeks.

Hormonal changes will affect almost every organ in the body. Some signs of early pregnancy in many women include symptoms like:

- Extreme fatigue

- Tender, swollen breasts. Nipples may protrude.

- Nausea with or without vomiting (morning sickness)

- Cravings or aversion to certain foods

- Mood swings

- Constipation

- Frequent urination

- Headache

- Heartburn

- Weight gain or loss

Revise your daily routine

Some of the changes you experience in your first trimester may cause you to revise your daily routine. You may need to go to bed earlier or eat more frequent or smaller meals.

Some women experience a lot of discomfort, and others may not feel any at all. Pregnant women experience pregnancy differently and even if they've been pregnant before. Pregnant women may feel completely differently with each subsequent pregnancy.

CHANGES IN THE SECOND TRIMESTER: WEEK 13 – WEEK 28

Changes a Woman May Experience:

Once you enter the second trimester you may find it easier than the first. Your nausea (morning sickness) and fatigue may lessen or go away completely. However, you will also notice more changes in your body. That **"baby bump"** will start to show as your abdomen expands with the growing baby. By the end of the second trimester you will even be able to feel your baby move!

Physical changes in the second trimester:

Some changes you may notice in your body in the second trimester include:

- Back, abdomen, groin, or thigh aches and pains

- **Stretch marks** on your abdomen, breasts, thighs, or buttocks

- Darkening of the skin around your nipples

- A line on the skin running from belly button to pubic hairline (**linea nigra**)

- Patches of darker skin, usually over the cheeks, forehead, nose, or upper lip. This is sometimes called the mask of pregnancy (**Melasma,** or **Chloasma facies**).

- Numb or tingling hands (**carpal tunnel syndrome**)

- Itching on the abdomen, palms, and soles of the feet. *(Call your doctor if you have nausea, loss of appetite, vomiting, yellowing of skin, or fatigue combined with itching. These can be **signs of a liver problem.**)*

- Swelling of the ankles, fingers, and face. *(**If you notice any sudden or extreme swelling or if you gain a lot of weight quickly, call your doctor immediately.** This could be a **sign of a serious condition** called **preeclampsia**.)*

CHANGES IN THIRD TRIMESTER: WEEK 29 – WEEK 40 (BIRTH)

Changes a Woman May Experience:

The third trimester is the final stage of pregnancy. Discomforts that started in the second trimester will likely continue, along with some new ones.

As the baby grows and puts more pressure on your internal organs, you may find you have difficulty breathing and have to urinate more frequently. This is normal and once you give birth, these problems should disappear.

You will notice more physical changes, including:

- Swelling of the ankles, fingers, and face. *(If you notice any sudden or extreme swelling or if you gain a lot of weight really quickly, consult your doctor right away. This could be a sign of a serious condition called preeclampsia.)*

- Haemorrhoids.

- Tender breasts, which may leak a watery pre-milk called colostrum

- Your belly button may protrude

- The baby **"dropping,"** or moving lower in your abdomen

- Contractions, which can be a sign of real or false labour.

- Other symptoms you may notice in the third trimester include shortness of breath, heartburn, and difficulty sleeping.

Changes that you can't see:

Other changes are happening in your body during the third trimester that you can't see.

As your due date approaches, your cervix becomes thinner and softer in a process called effacement that helps the cervix open during childbirth. Your doctor will monitor the progress of your pregnancy with regular exams, especially as you near your due date.

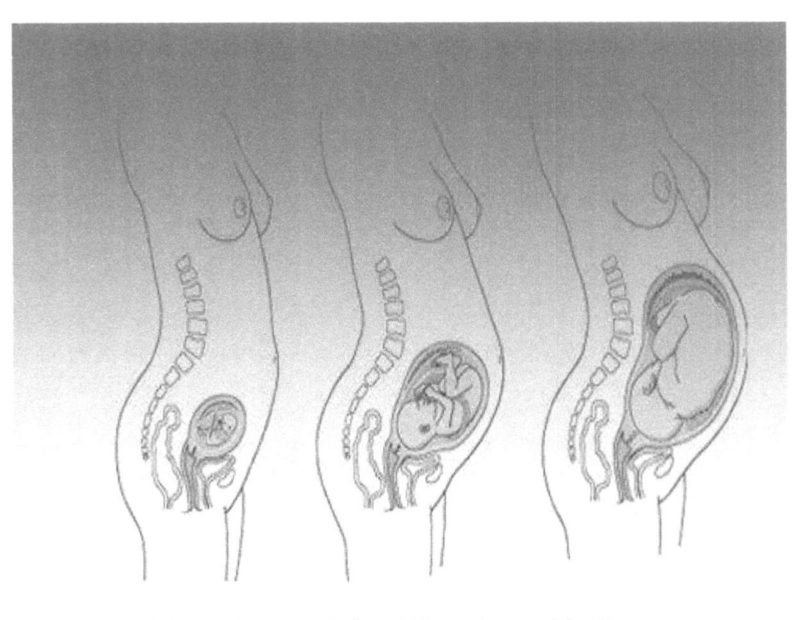

First Trimester
Second Trimester
Third Trimester

CHAPTER: 7

GROWTH AND DEVELOPMENT OF EMBRYO/FOETUS - WEEK BY WEEK

The development of an embryo during the initial eight weeks of pregnancy is a remarkable and rapid process.

Some key changes that occur during this period:

Week-1

- **Fertilization:** Union of the sperm and egg.

- **Formation of Zygote:** The fertilized egg divides rapidly as it travels down the fallopian tube toward the uterus.

Week 2

- **Formation of blastocyst:** The zygote becomes a blastocyst, a hollow ball of cells.

- **Implantation:** The blastocyst attaches to the uterine lining.

Week 3

- **Formation of germ layers:** Ectoderm, mesoderm, and endoderm—the fundamental layers—begin to form.

- **Development of neural tubes:** The basis for the nervous system develops.

Week 4

- **Organogenesis:** Organs begin to form from the three germ layers.

- **Heart Development:** The heart starts to beat

- **Limbs begin to bud:** Arm and leg buds start to appear

Week 5

- **Formation of major organs:** Organs such as the brain, spinal cord, heart, and gastrointestinal tract continue to develop.

- **Formation of eyes and ears:** Basic structures of eyes and ears become visible.

Week 6

- **Brain Development:** The brain continues to develop rapidly.

- **Limb formation:** Paddle-like hands and feet begin to form.

- **Nose and mouth formation:** Basic structures of the face start to appear.

Week 7

- **Developing facial features:** Eyes become more distinct, and facial features continue to develop.

- **Formation of fingers and toes:** Hand and foot plates separate into fingers and toes.

Week 8

Refinement of organs: Hand and foot plates separate into fingers and toes.

External genitalia differentiation: Differentiation of male and female external genitalia starts.

These weeks are vital for the embryo's development, with the formation of major organ systems and the establishment of the basic body plan. It's during this time that any disruptions or adverse   influences can significantly impact the embryo's development.

Weeks 1 to 8

- The egg is fertilized by sperm and a growing ball of cells called the blastocyst implants in the uterus.

- Week 5 begins the embryo stage of development.

- The brain and spine begin to form, followed by the neural tube.

- Cardiac tissue starts to develop.

- Parts of the face take shape and the inner ear begins to develop.

- Arm and leg buds appear, and then webbed fingers and toes emerge.

- The long tube that will become the digestive tract takes shape. By the end of week 8, the embryo is about half an inch long.

Week 9

During the 9th to 12th weeks of pregnancy, the embryo continues its rapid development, transitioning into a foetus.

- **Foetal stage:** The embryo is now officially referred to as a foetus.

- **Rapid growth:** The foetus experiences a rapid growth phase.

- **Refinement of organs:** Organs continue to mature and refine their structures.

- **Formation of joints:** Limb movements become more coordinated as joints form.

Week 10

- **Development of bones:** Cartilage starts to harden into bone.

- **Facial features:** The face becomes more human-like, with distinct facial features.

- **Movement:** The fetus starts making small movements, though not yet felt by the mother.

Week 11

- **Development of reproductive organs:** The fetus develops its reproductive organs, though they are not yet distinguishable externally.

- **Digestive system maturation:** The digestive system further develops.

- **Refinement of facial features:** The face becomes more defined.

Week 12

- **External genitalia:** External genitalia become more differentiated and may be visible through ultrasound.

- **Muscle development:** Muscles continue to develop, allowing for more coordinated movements.

- **Formation of reflexes:** The foetus may start exhibiting reflex movements like sucking and swallowing.

- **By the end of week 12**, the fetus is about 2 inches long and weighs about half an ounce.

By the end of the 12th week, the most critical period of foetal development, the major organ systems are usually formed, although they will continue to mature and grow throughout the remainder of the pregnancy.

At this point, the risk of certain developmental issues decreases, though not entirely eliminated.

Week 13

- **Growth spurt:** The foetus experiences significant growth, doubling in size, compared to the previous weeks.

- **Movement:** The foetus begins to move more actively, although these movements are still not typically felt by the mother.

- **Vocal cord development:** Vocal cords begin to form

Week 14

- **Body Proportions:** The body starts to elongate, and the head becomes more proportional to the body.

- **Facial expressions:** The can make facial expressions, like squinting and frowning

- **Urine production:** The foetus starts producing urine, which is released into the amniotic fluid.

Week 15

- **Limb proportions:** Limbs continue to lengthen and become more proportionate

- **Hair and skin Development:** Fine hair called lanugo begins to cover the body and the skin becomes less transparent.

- **Fingerprints form:** unique fingerprints start to develop.

Week 16

- **Bone marrow formation:** Bone marrow starts to produce blood cells.

- **Sensory organs development:** Eyes and ears move closer to their final positions, and taste buds begin to form on the tongue.

- **Muscle Development:** Muscles continue to strengthen, allowing for more coordinated movements.

By the end of week 16, the foetus is more than 4 inches long and weighs more than 3 ounces and the foetus has developed many of its basic physiological structures and systems. While it is still in the early stages of development, the foetus is becoming more recognizable as a human being. The mother may also start feeling the first subtle movements of the foetus, commonly known as **"quickening."**

Week 17

- The foetus is about 5 inches long and around 5 ounces

- Cartilage starts to harden into bone

- The umbilical cord continues to grow stronger and thicker.

- The baby's movements become more coordinated, though they might not be   felt by the mother yet.

- The baby's facial features become more defined, and the skeleton continues to develop.

Week 18

- The part of the brain that controls motor movements is fully formed.

- The digestive system is working.

- The baby's weight increases to around 6.7 ounces.

- Fine hair called lanugo starts to cover the baby's body for warmth.

- Vernix caseosa begins to form on the skin, protecting it from the amniotic fluid

- The baby's ears move to their final position on the sides of the head. The foetus can hear sounds.

Week 19

- The foetus is about 6 inches long and weighs approximately 8.5 cms.

- Eyebrows and eyelashes start to grow

- The baby's movements become more pronounced, but they might still not be felt by the mother, especially if it is the first pregnancy.

- The skin becomes less translucent as fat stores begin to develop underneath.

Week 20

- The foetus is about 6-7 inches long and weighs around 10.5 ounces

- The mother might start feeling the baby's movements, known as quickening

- The baby's digestive system continues to mature and meconium, the baby's first bowel movement, starts to form in the intestines.

- The baby begins to regulate its temperature more effectively with the development of sweat glands.

- The sex of the baby might be identifiable through ultrasound as sexual characteristics become more distinct.

- During these weeks, the foetus undergoes significant growth and development as various organs and body systems continue to mature in preparation for birth.

- By the end of week 20, the fetus is more than 6 inches long and weighs less than 11 ounces.

Week 21

- The foetus measures about 10.5 inches and weighs approximately 12.7 ounces.

- Eyebrows and eyelids are more defined, and the baby's movements become more coordinated.

- The brain and nervous system continue to develop, enabling more complex movements and sensory experiences.

- The foetus's kicks and turns are stronger now.

- If the hand floats to the mouth, the foetus may suck its thumb.

- Eyebrows are visible.

Week 22

- The brain and nervous system continue to develop, enabling more complex movements and sensory experiences.

- The skin is still translucent but is gradually becoming less transparent as fat stores develop.

- The baby's organs, including the lungs, pancreas, and reproductive organs, continue to mature

Week 23

- The foetus measures about 11.5 inches and weighs roughly 1.1 pounds.

- Lung development accelerates, with the formation of air sacs that will eventually allow the baby to breathe air.

- The baby's skin is wrinkled and covered with vernix and lanugo to protect it and regulate temperature.

- At week 23, most of the foetus's sleep time is spent in rapid eye movements (REM) sleep.

- Ridges are forming in the hands and feet that later will be fingerprints and footprints.

Week 24

- The foetus measures around 12 inches and weighs approximately 1.3 pounds.

- The baby's brain continues to grow and develop rapidly, forming more   complex structures.

- Eyebrows and eyelashes are well-defined, and the foetus is gaining more body fat.

- The foetus's kicks and turns are stronger now.

- If the hand floats to the mouth, the fetus may suck its thumb.

- Eyebrows are visible.

During these weeks, the foetus experiences substantial growth and development, with organs maturing further in preparation for life outside the womb.

The baby's movements become more pronounced and may be felt more regularly by the mother, contributing to the bonding experience between parent and child.

Week 25

- The foetus measures about 13.5 inches in length and weighs around 1.5 pounds.

- Lungs continue developing, producing surfactant, a substance that helps the air sacs inflate easily.

- The baby's skin becomes less wrinkled due to the deposition of more fat under the skin

- The eyes begin to open, though they will still be used shut mostly until later.

Week 26

- The foetus measures approximately 14 inches and weighs about 1.7 pounds.

- The lungs continue maturing, and the baby starts practicing breathing movements by inhaling and exhaling amniotic fluid.

- The lungs begin making surfactant, a substance needed for breathing after birth

- The brain is rapidly developing, with increasing activity in neural connections.

- The foetus can respond with movement to familiar sounds, such as your voice.

- Loud sounds may make the foetus respond by pulling in arms and legs.

Week 27

- The foetus measures around 14.4 inches and weighs roughly 2 pounds.

- The baby's lungs are still developing, but survival outside the womb becomes   increasingly possible with medical advancement.

- Eyes are open, and the baby starts responding to light and sound stimuli.

- At 27 weeks, more fat is being added to keep the foetus warm.

- A greasy material called vernix has started to develop. Vernix acts as a   waterproof barrier that protects the skin

Week 28:

- The foetus measures about 14.8 inches and weighs approximately 2.2 pounds

- Rapid brain development continues, allowing for more complex brain functions.

- The baby's body begins to fill out as fat stores increase for insulation and energy.

Week 29:

- The foetus measures around 15.2 inches and weighs about 2.5 pounds.

- The baby's muscles and lungs continue to mature, and breathing movements become more coordinate.

- The bones are hardening, but they are still relatively flexible to ease the birthing process.

Week 30:

- The foetus measures approximately 15.7 inches and weighs around 3 pounds.

- Brain development continues at a rapid pace, enabling the baby to regulate body temperature more effectively.

- The baby's fingernails and toenails are fully formed.

- During these weeks, the foetus experiences significant growth and development, with major organ systems continuing to mature in preparation for birth.

- The baby becomes more responsive to external stimuli, and vital organs like the lungs continue to mature, making survival outside the womb increasingly feasible, albeit with potential medical assistance if born prematurely

Week 32

- The foetus can stretch, kick, and make grasping motions.

- The eyes can open and close and sense changes in light.

- The bone marrow is forming red blood cells.

- At week 31, major development is finished, and the foetus is gaining weight very quickly.

- In boys, the testicles have begun to descend into the scrotum.

- At week 32, the fine hair that covered the foetus's body (lanugo) begins to disappear.

- By the end of week 32, the foetus is almost 17 inches long and weighs a little more than 4 pounds.

Month 9-Weeks 33 to 36

- The brain is growing and developing rapidly.

- The bones harden, but the skull remains soft and flexible.

- More fat is forming under the skin.

- The fingernails have grown to the ends of the fingers.

- During week 36 or 37, most foetuses turn to a head-down position for birth.

- By the end of week 36, the foetus is about 18 inches long and weighs a little more than 6 pounds.

Month 10

Weeks 37 to 40

- The lungs, brain, and nervous system continue to Develop.

- The circulatory system is complete, and so is the Musculo-skeletal system.

- The foetus is taking up a lot of space in the amniotic sac and you should continue to feel movements.

- By now, the foetus's head may have dropped lower into position in your pelvis.

- By the end of week 40, the foetus is 20 inches long and may weigh 7½ to 8 pounds.

- Average birth weight is between 6 pounds 2 ounces to 9 pounds 2 ounces and average length is 19 to 21 inches long. Most full-term babies fall within these ranges, but healthy babies come in many different weights and sizes.

CHAPTER: 8

EMOTIONAL AND HORMONAL CHANGES DURING PREGNANCY

YOUR FEELINGS AND EMOTIONS DURING PREGNANCY

Pregnancy might leave you feeling **delighted, anxious, exhilarated** and **exhausted** — sometimes all at once. Even if you're thrilled about being pregnant, a new baby adds **emotional stress** to your life.

It's natural for you to worry about your baby's health, your adjustment to parenthood and the financial demands of raising a child. If you are working, you might worry about how to balance the demands of family and career.

You might also experience mood swings.

What you are feeling is normal.

During pregnancy you will probably feel many ups and downs. You may experience some or all of these emotions (and they may change quickly):

- **Surprise** – if your pregnancy is unexpected. You may then feel joy (if you welcome the pregnancy) or fear (if you are unsure about the change to your life) or both.

- **Happiness** – particularly if you have been **trying to have a baby** and you feel well.

- **Anger** – which can result from your body's hormonal changes, from a sense of being vulnerable, or from pregnancy symptoms that are uncomfortable or painful.

- **Fear for the baby's health** – if you have concerns about your baby having an illness or disability. If you are worried about a particular risk, talk to your midwife or doctor.

- **Fear of birth** – which is a recognised psychological disorder. Counselling and talking with your midwife or doctor can help you overcome this fear.

- **Love** – for your baby, your partner and your family.

- **Sadness or disappointment** – if you have illness or complications during your pregnancy, or you can't have the birth plan that you would prefer.

- **General sadness about the world** – whereby you find it hard to watch the news or hear sad stories about children or families.

- **Grief** – if you suffer a **miscarriage**, a loss at a later stage of pregnancy, or a stillbirth.

- **Prolonged sadness from perinatal depression** – in this case, you will need the help of mental health specialists.

MOOD SWINGS DURING PREGNANCY

The hormones changing in your body mean you will probably have heightened emotions, both positive and negative. And you will probably swing between these emotions. **While you may be overjoyed about having a baby, you may also be stressed and overwhelmed. You may feel worried about whether:**

- your baby will affect your relationship with your partner

- you will cope financially

- you will be able to juggle work and parenting

- you will be a good mother

- the baby will be healthy

- your other children will accept and love the new baby.

You may also feel unimpressed with your changing body. You may be worried about putting on too much weight, or not enough. Or not being able to do the physical activity that you usually do. Or not looking attractive to your partner. Add the hormone-induced **fatigue, forgetfulness and moodiness**, and you may feel completely out of control. **This is all common.**

WAYS TO COPE WITH PREGNANCY EMOTIONS

While it may seem overwhelming, there are many things you can do to cope and make your emotions more manageable.

- **Self-care**: Listen to your body and mind and be aware of what you need. If a bubble bath sounds relaxing, do it. If you need time alone to relax and read a book or get a pedicure, make time for it.

- **Sleep**: Getting 8 hours of good sleep can do amazing things for your emotional state. While this may not always be possible, do everything you can to get a healthy amount of sleep. You can experiment with sleeping positions, let your partner know if you are having difficulty sleeping so the two of you can come up with a plan to make sure you are getting the sleep you need.

- **Diet**: Like sleep, what you eat is a great natural way to help with your mood and emotions. Eating healthy and natural foods, instead of processed foods, promotes both physical and mental health, which contributes to increased emotional stability.

- **Support**: A supportive and encouraging group of people surrounding you is incredibly important during pregnancy. Making close family and friends aware of your emotions and having people to talk to when you feel overwhelmed is extremely helpful for your emotional health. In some cases, if you are having difficulty with your emotions, professional counselling may be an option to explore.

Pregnancy can be a beautiful time, but it is important to be prepared for the changes that may occur in your emotional state. It is important to remember pregnancy emotions are normal and not to feel guilty for the array of emotions you are feeling but to be aware of them and respond in a healthy, positive way. Let your doctor know if you feel like your emotions are extremely unstable, you are experiencing severe depression, or having thoughts of suicide. In these cases, medical intervention or professional counselling may be necessary.

You should take care of yourself, and look to loved ones for understanding and encouragement. If your mood changes become severe or intense, you should consult your health care provider. Your health care provider will treat, educate and reassure you throughout your pregnancy.

Your first visit will focus on assessing your overall health, identifying any risk factors and determining your baby's gestational age. Your health care provider will ask detailed questions about your health history. You should be honest. If you are uncomfortable discussing your health history in front of your partner, schedule a private consultation. Also you should expect to learn about first trimester screening for chromosomal abnormalities.

HORMONAL CHANGES DURING PREGNANCY

During pregnancy, a variety of hormones play crucial roles in supporting and regulating the growth and development of the foetus. Some of the key hormones involved include:

1. Progesterone: Progesterone is produced by the ovaries and placenta, and it helps to prepare the uterus for implantation of the fertilized egg. It also helps to maintain the pregnancy by preventing contractions of the uterus.

2. Oestrogen: Oestrogen is produced by the ovaries and placenta, and it stimulates the growth of the uterus and placenta. It also helps to increase blood flow to the uterus, which provides nutrients to the developing foetus.

3. Human chorionic gonadotropin (HCG): HCG is produced by the placenta and is the hormone that is detected in a pregnancy test. It helps to maintain the pregnancy by preventing ovulation and by stimulating the production of progesterone.

These hormones play complex and interrelated roles in regulating the pregnancy, and imbalances or changes in their levels can indicate potential problems. For example, **low levels of HCG** can indicate a potential **miscarriage**, while **high levels of oestrogen** can indicate an **increased risk of preeclampsia,** a pregnancy-related condition that causes high blood pressure and damage to organs.

It's important for pregnant women to work closely with their healthcare provider to monitor these hormone levels and ensure a healthy pregnancy.

PLACENTAL FUNCTION

The placenta is a specialized organ that forms during pregnancy to provide essential nutrients and oxygen to the growing foetus. It also acts as a barrier to prevent harmful substances, such as drugs and toxins, from reaching the foetus. Some of the key functions of the placenta include:

1. Nutrient exchange: The placenta acts as an interface between the mother's blood supply and the foetal blood supply, allowing for the exchange of nutrients, oxygen, and waste products.

2. Hormonal regulation: The placenta produces hormones, such as oestrogen and human chorionic gonadotropin (HCG) that play important roles in maintaining the pregnancy and supporting foetal growth and development

3. Waste removal: The placenta helps to remove waste products, such as carbon dioxide and urea, from the foetus, and ensures that the foetus has a clean supply of blood.

4. Protection from harmful substances: The placenta acts as a barrier to prevent harmful substances, such as drugs and toxins, from reaching the foetus, protecting it from harm.

The placenta is a vital component of a healthy pregnancy, and it plays a critical role in ensuring that the foetus has the necessary resources for growth and development.

CHAPTER: 9

ANTENATAL CARE

What is Antenatal Care and why is it Necessary?

Antenatal care (also called **prenatal care**) is the care and monitoring of a pregnant woman and her developing foetus during pregnancy. The goal of antenatal care is to promote a healthy pregnancy and delivery, and to prevent or detect and treat any potential problems that may arise during pregnancy. Antenatal care typically includes regular prenatal visits with a healthcare provider, who will assess the health of the woman and the developing foetus. During these visits, the provider may perform a physical examination, order laboratory tests, and perform ultrasound scans to monitor foetal growth and development.

Antenatal care is the care of the woman during pregnancy to achieve a healthy mother and a healthy baby. Pregnancy, Labor and birth of a child are important milestones in a couple's life. Regular medical care, knowledge of your choices, and understanding the unknown events during pregnancy can make childbirth an extremely enriching and joyful event.

Objectives:

- To reduce maternal and infant mortality and morbidity

- Early detection of high risk cases and management

- Timely detection and management of complications

- Ensure the birth of a healthy child

- Ensure the health of the mother

- Provide essential health education to the Pregnant woman

Goals:

- Early, accurate estimation of gestational age

- Identification of pregnancies at increased risk for maternal or foetal morbidity and mortality

- On-going evaluation of maternal and foetal health status

- Anticipation of problems with intervention, if possible, to prevent or minimize morbidity

- Health promotion, education, support, and shared decision making

FREQUENCY OF ANTENATAL VISITS

- Booking visit: to be at 6 weeks of gestation

- 6th to 28th week : every 4 weeks

- 29th to 36th week- every 2 weeks

- 36th week to up to delivery-every week

More frequent visits- if there are abnormalities or complications or danger signs arise during pregnancy

ANTENATAL CARE COMPRISES

1. Registration of Pregnancy

2. History taking

3. Antenatal examination-General and obstetrical

4. Laboratory Investigations

5. Health education

PHYSICAL EXAMINATION

1. Weight

- At the time of registration baseline weight

- Normal weight gain in pregnancy- 9-11 Kgs.

- After the 1st trimester 0.5 Kg weight per week

- Low weight gain --Intrauterine growth restriction of the foetus.

- Excessive weight gain –Preeclampsia, Twins, Hydramnios.

2. **Blood pressure:** High B.P.(.140/90mm.hg.) indicates preeclampsia

3. **Pallor:** Indicate anaemia. Identified by seeing the lower palpebral conjunctiva, tongue, oral mucosa, palms and nails

4. **Respiratory rate:** More than 33 R.R./minute and pallor indicates severe anaemia

5. **Generalised oedema and puffiness of face:** Indicates preeclampsia

6. **Abdominal examination:** Progress of pregnancy/ foetal growth /foetal lie and presentation is Known, Foetal heart sounds are heard.

An unexpectedly **large uterus** indicates wrong date of LMP/full bladder./ multiple pregnancy/ polyhydramnios / hydatidiform mole/ pregnancy with a pelvic tumor and

A **small for dates uterus** indicates wrong dates of LMP / intrauterine growth restriction of the baby/ Missed abortion/IUD/ Transverse lie

INVESTIGATIONS: LAB AND ULTRASOUND

Lab:

1. **Routine tests:** The following lab tests are done early in pregnancy:

Blood

- Complete blood count (CBC) ,

- Blood Group & Rh type,

- Blood sugar

- TSH

- Rubella

- Hepatitis B –HBSAg

- Sexually transmitted infections (STIs)-VDRL,

- Human immunodeficiency virus (HIV),

- HCV

Urinalysis

- Complete urine examination

- Urine culture and sensitivity test

- Urine for Chlamydia and gonorrhoea identification

ULTRASOUND

Early pregnancy scan

Reasons for having an Early Pregnancy Scan are to:

- Rule out ectopic pregnancy and check whether the pregnancy sac is located within the uterus

- Confirm viability of pregnancy

- Check if there is a heartbeat.

- Calculate the gestation of pregnancy (number of weeks)

- Determine whether it is a singleton or multiple pregnancy

- Bleeding/Spotting or any unusual pain

ANOMALY SCAN - 1

FOETAL NUCHAL TRANSLUCENCY TEST (NT)

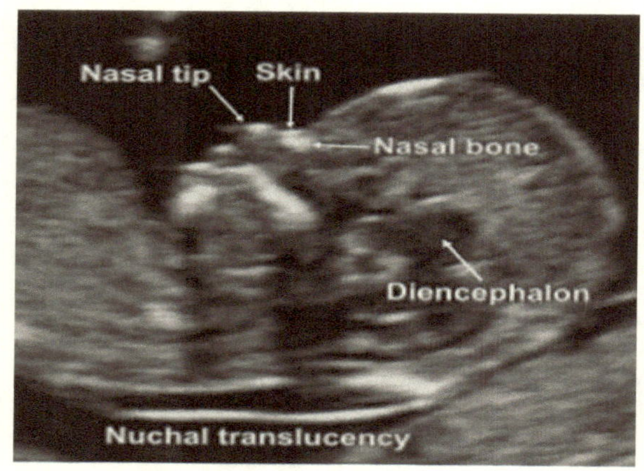

- Screening to detect chromosomal abnormality.

- The nuchal translucency scan (also called the NT scan) is to assess your developing baby's risk of having **Down syndrome (DS)** and some other chromosomal abnormalities, as well as **major congenital heart problems.**

- The NT scan measures the clear (translucent) space in the tissue at the back of your baby's neck.

- Babies with abnormalities tend to accumulate more fluid at the back of their neck during the first trimester, causing this clear space to be larger than average.

- The NT scan must be done when you're between 11 and 14 weeks pregnant, because this is when the base of your baby's neck is still transparent.

- Normally **NT** is less than 2 .5 mm. in the 1st trimester.

Foetal anomaly scan or Targeted Imaging For etal Anomalies (TIFFA) scan:

- Ultrasound is the main diagnostic tool in the prenatal detection of congenital abnormalities.

- It allows examination of the external and internal anatomy of the foetus and the detection of not only major defects but also of subtle markers of chromosomal abnormalities and genetic syndromes.

- Although some women are at high risk of fetal abnormalities, either because of a **family history** or due to **exposure to teratogens** such as **infection** and **various drugs**, the vast majority of fetal abnormalities occur in the low-risk group.

- Consequently, ultrasound examination should be offered routinely to all pregnant women.

- The scan, which is usually performed at **18–23 weeks of pregnancy**, should be carried out to a high standard and should include systematic examination of the foetus for the detection of both major and minor defects.

SCREENING TESTS

(Double marker, Triple marker & quadruple test) :

Done to analyse how likely an unborn baby is to have certain genetic disorders.

Double Marker Test :

- Free **βhCG** (human chorionic gonadotropin) and **PAPPA** (Pregnancy associated plasma protein A).

- **Free βhCG** is a glycoprotein hormone produced by the placenta during pregnancy. High level of this hormone is indicative to a higher risk of **Trisomy 18** and **Down's syndrome.**

- The **PAPP-A** and **βhCG** tests must be taken between **9 and 13 weeks gestation** (ideally between **10 and 12 weeks)**

- **NT scan carried out after 11** and **before 14 weeks gestation**.

Triple Marker test :

- This test is highly beneficial for women who are above the age of 35.

- Triple marker test is done to examine if there is any genetic disorder in the foetus or not

Some **genetic disorders** or **defects** include the following:

- Trisomy 18 or Edward's syndrome is a common type of chromosome abnormality.

- Down syndrome is a condition in which extra genetic material from chromosome 21 is included in the cell.

- Neural tube defects are congenital disabilities of the total nervous system, i.e., brain, spine, and spinal cord.

Who benefits from the triple marker test?

- Beneficial to women who are above the age of 35 or above.

- Couples who have a history of congenital disabilities. Women who use insulin and are diabetic patients can be satisfied with these test results. It helps to determine whether the baby is affected or not.

- **Triple marker test** is also helpful to those who have been highly exposed to radiation.

- Women having severe viral infection during pregnancy can also opt for this test but with a doctor's consultation.

Tests:

- AFP : alpha-fetoprotein is a protein that is produced by the foetus

- Free Beta hCG

- Estriol.

The usual range of triple marker test

- The average levels of triple screen markers in pregnant women ranged from 1.38 to 187.00 IU/ml for **AFP,** 1.06 to 315 ng/ml for β hCG, and from 0.25 to 28.5 nmol/l for **uE3.**

- Negative screen results indicate that the fetus is very low or not at risk of developing any congenital disabilities.

Quadruple Marker tests :

2nd Trimester screening : 14-16 weeks

- Free Beta HCG,

- AFP,

- E3,

- INHIBIN-A

CHAPTER: 10

UNDERSTAND THE ROUTINE TESTS DURING PREGNANCY

What tests are done early in pregnancy?

- Urinalysis

- Urine culture

- Urine-Screening for chlamydia and Gonorrhoea

- Complete blood count (CBC)

- Blood type and Rh factor

Tests for specific diseases and infections early in pregnancy, including:

- Rubella

- Hepatitis B and hepatitis C

- Human immunodeficiency virus (HIV)

- Other sexually transmitted infections (STIs)

- Tuberculosis (TB)

What is a urinalysis?

A urinalysis is a quick **test of your urine for**

- **Red blood cells**, a possible sign of a urinary tract disease

- **White blood cells,** a possible sign of a urinary tract infection (UTI)

- **Glucose,** because high levels of blood sugar can be a sign of diabetes mellitus

- This test also measures the amount of protein in your blood, which can be compared to levels later in pregnancy.

- High protein levels may signal kidney disease or preeclampsia, a serious complication that can occur later in pregnancy or after the baby is born.

What is a urine culture?

This test looks for bacteria in your urine, which can be a sign of a UTI. This test is done because sometimes UTIs do not cause symptoms (**Asymptomatic Bacteriuria**).

If the test shows bacteria in your urine, you should be treated with antibiotics. Repeat test after you finish treatment.

Why screen for Chlamydia and gonorrhoea?

Chlamydia and gonorrhoea can result in serious health complications if left untreated, including **spontaneous abortion, stillbirth, infant death in the first week of life, preterm delivery, and low birth weight**.

Both chlamydia and gonorrhoea **can be transmitted to babies during childbirth**, which can cause babies to later develop **conjunctivitis** (an eye infection) in the case of **gonorrhoea**, and conjunctivitis and/ or **pneumonia** in the case of **chlamydia.**

Urine sample or a vaginal or cervical swab can be used for screening. During pregnancy urine sample is preferred.

What does a complete blood count test for?

A CBC counts the number of different types of cells that make up your blood. The number of **red blood cells** can show whether you have a certain type of **anaemia**. The number of **white blood cells** can show how many **disease-fighting cells** are in your blood. The number of **platelets** can reveal whether you have a problem with **blood clotting.**

Will I be tested for blood type?

Yes, during the first trimester of pregnancy you will have a blood test to find out your blood type, such as type A or type B. Also, your blood will be tested for the **Rh factor.**

What is the Rh factor?

The Rh factor is a protein that can be found on the surface of red blood cells. If your blood cells have this protein, you are Rh positive. If your blood cells do not have this protein, you are Rh negative. The **"positive"** or

"negative" part of your blood type, such as **O positive** or **A negative**, refers to your Rh status.

Why is it important to know your Rh status?

If you are Rh negative and your foetus is Rh positive, your body can make antibodies against the Rh factor.

These antibodies can damage the foetus's red blood cells. This usually does not cause problems in a first pregnancy, when your body makes only a small number of antibodies. But it can cause serious issues in a later pregnancy, including stillbirth.

What will happen if I am Rh negative?

If you are Rh negative, you may be given medication during pregnancy to help prevent the development of Rh antibodies. If you are Rh negative and have already made a certain number of Rh antibodies, you might need special tests and monitoring throughout pregnancy. Your baby may also need treatment after birth.

Why is testing for rubella done?

Rubella (sometimes called German measles) can **cause birth defects** if you are **infected during pregnancy.** Your blood can show whether you have been infected with rubella or if you have been vaccinated against this disease. If you had this infection before or you have been vaccinated against rubella, you are immune to the disease.

What if I'm not immune to rubella?

Rubella is easily spread. If your blood test shows you are not immune, avoid anyone who has the disease while you are pregnant. There is a vaccine, but it contains a live virus and is not recommended during pregnancy. You can get the measles-mumps-rubella (MMR) vaccine after the baby is born.

What is hepatitis?

Hepatitis is a virus that infects the liver. If you are pregnant and have **hepatitis B or hepatitis C, you can pass the virus to your foetus.** Everyone should be tested for hepatitis B and hepatitis C infection during pregnancy.

What if I have Hepatitis during pregnancy?

If you are infected with hepatitis B or hepatitis C, you might need special care during pregnancy. Your baby may also need special care after birth.

You can breastfeed if you have either infection. A **vaccine** is available to protect the baby against hepatitis B. The vaccine is given as a series of three shots, with the first dose given to the baby within a few hours of birth.

Why is it important to have a test for HIV?

HIV attacks cells of the body's immune system and causes acquired immunodeficiency syndrome (AIDS) if not treated. If you have HIV, there is a chance you could pass it to your foetus.

HIV during Pregnancy

While you are pregnant, you can take medication that can greatly reduce the risk of passing HIV to your foetus. You can also get specialized care to ensure that you stay as healthy as possible throughout your pregnancy. This is why everyone is tested for HIV early in pregnancy.

What other STI tests are done?

- Everyone is tested for **syphilis** early in pregnancy. You should also be tested for **chlamydia** and **gonorrhoea** if you are under age 25 or if you are at increased risk for getting STIs.

- These tests are done early in pregnancy because these infections can cause complications for you and your foetus. Tests for these infections may be repeated later in pregnancy based on your age and risk factors.

Syphilis, Chlamydia, Gonorrhoea in pregnancy

If you have syphilis, chlamydia, or gonorrhoea, you should be treated during pregnancy and tested again to see if the treatment has worked. Your sex partner or partners should also be treated to prevent you from getting infected again.

Who should be tested for TB?

People who are at high risk of TB should be tested for it. Those at high risk include people who are infected with

HIV, live in close contact with someone who has TB, or are from a country with high rates of TB.

Tests Done Later in Pregnancy

The tests done later in pregnancy **include glucose screening and group B streptococcus (GBS) screening.**

What is a glucose screening test?

This test measures the level of glucose, or sugar, in your blood. A high blood sugar level may be a sign of gestational diabetes, which can cause problems during pregnancy. For this test, you drink a special sugar mixture. An hour later, a blood sample is taken and sent to a lab. If your blood sugar level is high, you should have another type of glucose test to confirm the results.

When is a glucose screening done?

This test usually is done between **24 and 28 weeks of pregnancy**. This test might be done in the first trimester of pregnancy if you have risk factors for diabetes or had gestational diabetes in a past pregnancy.

Genetic Testing for Birth Defects

What is the first step to screen for birth defects during pregnancy?

Screening for birth defects begins by assessing your risk factors. If you do have risk factors, you might want to see a genetic counsellor for more detailed information about your risks

What factors increase the risk of birth defects?

Most babies with birth defects are born to couples without risk factors. But the risk of birth defects is higher when certain factors are present. Risk factors include:

- Having a personal or family history of birth defects

- Belonging to certain ethnic groups

- Being 35 or older

- Having diabetes before pregnancy

What is the difference between screening and diagnostic testing for birth defects?

When done during pregnancy, screening tests can tell you the chances that the foetus may be at risk for certain common birth defects. A screening test cannot tell whether the foetus actually has a birth defect. There is **no risk to the foetus from screening tests.**

Diagnostic tests can **detect many, but not all, birth defects** caused by defects in a gene or chromosomes. You can choose to have diagnostic tests instead of or in addition to screening tests. **Some diagnostic tests carry risks**, including a small risk of **pregnancy loss.**

Am I required to have screening or testing for birth defects?

No, screening and testing are a personal choice. Knowing beforehand allows the option of deciding not to continue the pregnancy. If you choose to continue the pregnancy, knowing beforehand gives you time to prepare for having a child with a disorder. This means you can organize the medical care your child may need. Talk with your ob-gyn or genetic counsellor about your test results.

CHAPTER: 11

OVER VIEW OF YOUR PREGNANCY CARE

Blossoming Beginnings: Navigating the Journey of Pregnancy

BEFORE YOU GET PREGNANT

Think about the lifestyle factors that might affect your ability to conceive pregnancy and have a healthy pregnancy. Chances are more to get pregnant if you and your partner, both are in good health.

- Eat a balanced diet.

- Maintain a healthy weight.

- You should avoid drinking alcohol and quit smoking if you are trying to conceive. Or pregnant

- Regular exercise.

- If you or your partner takes any medication, consult your doctor and enquire whether it will affect your pregnancy.

- Take 400 micrograms of folic acid a day. You should continue to take this until you are 12 weeks pregnant.

- If you already have a baby with spina bifida or neural tube defects, or if you have coeliac disease, diabetes, are obese or take anti-epileptic medicines, ask your health care provider for more advice.

- If you have a health problem like mental health problems, diabetes or a family history of any hereditary diseases, talk to your doctor or a specialist before conception

AFTER YOU GET PREGNANT

0–8 weeks

- Soon after you are pregnant, consult your doctor to have advice for proper antenatal care.

- Some pregnant women start to feel sick or tired or have other minor physical problems for a few weeks.

- If you are not already taking folic acid supplements, you should start now.

8-12 weeks

- At your first visit, your weight, height and body mass index will be measured.

- You will be asked about your health and family history as well as husband's family history.

- You will be offered blood tests for Complete blood picture, Thyroid profile, Blood sugar, Vit.D, hepatitis B, HCV, HIV, VDRL and rubella.

- Ultrasound scan - This will check the site of pregnancy, single or multiple pregnancy, foetal heart rate and the baby's measurements and give an accurate due date.

- Your midwife will also discuss the whooping cough and flu vaccines which are offered to all pregnant women and your flu vaccine will be given at any stage of your pregnancy during flu season.

- Make a dental appointment.

- Just 12 weeks after conception, your baby is fully formed. It has all its organs, muscles, limbs and bones, and its sex organs are well developed.

- Your baby is already moving about but you cannot feel the movements yet.

12–16 weeks

- Find out about antenatal education, or antenatal awareness programs, including breast feeding.

- Make sure you are wearing a supportive bra. Your breasts will probably increase in size during pregnancy so you need to make sure you are wearing the right sized bra.

- If you have been feeling sick and tired, you will probably start to feel better around this time.

- You will be offered NT scan and Double marker test to detect foetal anomalies.

- Your pregnancy may just be beginning to show. This varies a lot from woman to woman.

16-20 weeks

- You may start to feel your baby move.

- Your tummy will begin to get bigger and you will need looser clothes.

- You may feel a surge of energy.

- Try to do your pregnancy exercises regularly

- Your midwife or doctor should:

    — review, discuss and record the results of any screening tests;

    — measure your blood pressure and test your urine for protein;

    — consider an iron supplement if you are anaemic.

- Your midwife or doctor should give you information about the anomaly scan and you will be offered at 18–20 weeks and answer any questions you have.

- Your baby is now growing quickly. Their face becomes much more defined and their hair, eyebrows and eyelashes are beginning to grow.

20-25 weeks

- Your uterus will begin to get bigger more quickly and you will really begin to look pregnant.

- You may feel hungrier than before. Stick to a sensible balanced diet

- You will begin to feel your baby move.

25 weeks

- Your baby is now moving around vigorously and responds to touch and sound.

- If this is your first baby, you will have an appointment with your midwife or doctor and they should:

  — check the size of your uterus

  — measure your blood pressure and

  — test your urine for protein.

28 weeks

- Your baby is now moving around vigorously and responds to touch and sound.

- Your midwife or doctor should check:

  — Blood pressure

  — urine for protein

  — the size of your uterus, foetal position and presentation and foetal heart sounds

31 weeks

Your midwife or doctor should:

— record Blood pressure

— check urine for protein

— check the size of your uterus, foetal position and presentation and foetal heart sounds

— review, discuss and record the results of any screening tests from the last appointment;

— scan and repeat blood tests done at the time of first visit

34 Weeks

• Your midwife or doctor will give you information about preparing for labour and birth.

— Inform you the symptoms and signs of active labour, ways of coping with pain in

— Labour and ways of structuring your birth plan.

— Review, record and discuss the results of any screening tests from the last appointment

— Measure the size of your uterus

— Measure your blood pressure and test your urine for protein.

- You may enquire about the availability of standard maternity facilities for birth.

- Get your bag ready if you are planning to give birth in hospital or in a midwifery unit.

- You will probably be attending antenatal classes now.

- You may be more aware of your uterus tightening from time to time. These are mild contractions known as Braxton Hicks contractions

- You may feel quite tired. Make sure you get plenty of rest.

36 weeks

Make sure you have all your important telephone numbers handy in case labour starts

- Your midwife or doctor should give you information about:

  — preparation of breasts for feeding the baby

  — feeding your baby;

  — caring for your new-born baby;

  — vitamin K and screening tests for your new-born baby

  — the 'baby blues' and postnatal depression.

- Your midwife or doctor should:

— measure the size of your uterus;

— check the position of your baby;

— measure your blood pressure and test your urine for protein.

- Sleeping may be increasingly difficult.

38 weeks

- Most women will go into labour spontaneously between 38 and 42 weeks.

- Your midwife or doctor should give you information about your options if your pregnancy lasts longer than 41 weeks.

- Your midwife or doctor should:

  — measure your blood pressure and

  — test your urine for protein.

  — measure the size of your uterus;

Call your hospital or midwife at any time if you have any worries about your baby or about labour and birth.

40 weeks

- Your midwife or doctor should give you more information about what happens if your pregnancy lasts longer than 41 weeks.

- Your midwife or doctor should:

- — measure your blood pressure

- — test your urine for protein.

- — measure the size of your uterus

41 weeks

- If your pregnancy lasts longer than 41 weeks, you may be induced. Your midwife or doctor will explain what this means and what the risks are.

- Your midwife or doctor should:

  - — measure the size of your uterus;

  - — measure your blood pressure

  - — test your urine for protein;

  - — offer a membrane sweep

  - — discuss your options and choices for induction of labour

CHAPTER: 12

COMMON DISCOMFORTS DURING PREGNANCY

Empowering Strategies for a More Comfortable Pregnancy Journey

Pregnancy, with its marvels and joys, often accompanies a range of **physical discomforts** that can vary widely among expectant mothers. Understanding and effectively managing these discomforts can significantly enhance the overall well-being and comfort of the mother-to-be.

PHYSICAL DISCOMFORTS DURING PREGNANCY

1. MORNING SICKNESS AND NAUSEA OR VOMITING

Nausea is very common in the early weeks of pregnancy , while your body is adjusting to the higher hormone levels and can happen any time during the day but may be worse in the morning, when your stomach is empty (that why it's called "morning sickness") or if you aren't eating enough.

Nausea and vomiting are not usually associated with a poor pregnancy outcome.

Recommendations:

- If nausea is a problem in the morning, eat dry foods like cereal, toast or crackers before getting out of bed.

- Try eating a high-protein snack such as lean meat or cheese before going to bed (protein takes longer to digest).

- Avoid sudden movements.

- Get out of bed slowly.

- Having regular small meals that are high in carbohydrate **can help to reduce morning sickness.**

- If you are hungry but extremely nauseated, **try the BRAT (bananas, rice and tea) diet.**

- Ginger may combat nausea.

- Eat small meals or snacks every two to three hours rather than three large meals.

- Eat   slowly and chew your food completely.

- Sip on fluids throughout the day. Avoid large amounts of fluids at one time. Try cool, clear fruit juices, such as apple or grape juice.

- Avoid spicy, fried, or greasy foods

- If you are bothered by strong smells, eat foods cold or at room temperature to minimize or avoid odours that bother you.

- Talk to your doctor about taking vitamin B6.

- Contact your health care provider if your vomiting is constant or so severe that you can't keep fluids or foods down. This can cause dehydration and should be treated right away.

- Breathe fresh air to help relieve nausea.

- It usually **disappears** around the **12ᵗʰ to 14ᵗʰ** week of your pregnancy.

2. FREQUENT URINATION

- Your growing uterus and baby press against your bladder, causing a frequent need to urinate during the **first trimester**.

- This will happen again in the **third trimester**, when the baby's head drops into the pelvis before birth.

Recommendations:

- Don't wear tight-fitting underwear, pants, or panty.

- If your urine burns or stings, it could be a sign of urinary tract infection. Contact your health care provider right away to treat it.

- Decrease fluid intake at night.

- Maintain fluid intake during day.

- Void when you feel the urge.

3. FATIGUE

- The body undergoes tremendous changes during pregnancy, leading to increased fatigue.

- Feeling tired might be because your growing baby requires extra energy. Sometimes, it's a sign of anaemia, which is common during pregnancy

Recommendations:

- Get plenty of rest; Rest frequently, Go to bed earlier and take naps.

- Keep a regular schedule when possible.

- Balance activity with rest. Moderate exercise daily boosts your energy level.

- If you think you may have anaemia, ask your health care provider to test your blood.

- Prioritizing activities and seeking support from partners or loved ones to manage household tasks can also conserve energy.

4. HEADACHES

Headaches can happen anytime during pregnancy. They can be caused by

- Tension,

- Congestion,

- Constipation, or in some cases,

- May be a ***sign of high blood pressure***, **preeclampsia.**

Recommendations:

- Put an ice pack on your forehead or the back of your neck.

- Rest, sit, or lie quietly in a low-lit room. Close your eyes and try to relax your back,   neck, and shoulders.

- Drugs like paracetamol or acetaminophen may help. But if your headaches don't subside, are severe, make you nauseous, or affect your vision, tell your doctor.

5. BLEEDING AND SWOLLEN GUMS

Your blood circulation and hormone levels can make your gums **tender** and **swollen**, and you may notice they **bleed more easily.**

Recommendations:

- Get a dental check -up early in your pregnancy to make sure your teeth and mouth are healthy.

- See your dentist if you notice a particular problem.

- Brush your teeth and floss regularly.

6. HEART BURN AND INDIGESTION

Hormonal changes can relax the valve between the stomach and oesophagus, leading to heartburn and indigestion.

Recommendations

- Eating smaller, more frequent meals

- Avoiding spicy or acidic foods.

- Remaining upright after meals

- Using pillows to prop oneself up while sleeping.

7. SWELLING IN THE FEET AND LEGS

Pressure from your growing uterus on the blood vessels carrying blood from the lower body causes fluid retention. The result is swelling (oedema) in the legs and feet.

Recommendations:

- Try not to stay on your feet for long periods of time. Avoid standing in one place.

- Drink plenty of fluids (at least 10-12 glasses of fluids a day).

- Avoid foods high in salt (sodium).

- Elevate your legs and feet while sitting. Avoid crossing your legs. Avoid tight stocking

- Wear loose, comfortable clothing; tight clothing can slow circulation and increase fluid retention.

- Don't wear tight shoes; choose supportive shoes with low, wide heels.

- Keep your diet rich in protein; too little protein can cause fluid reten.

- Notify your health care provider if your hands or face swell. This may be a warning sign of preeclampsia.

- Rest on your side during the day to help increase blood flow to your kidneys.

8. BREAST DISCOMFORTS

Breast Changes

- Most pregnant women will feel some changes in their breasts.

- Bluish veins may also appear as your blood supply increases.

- Your nipples can also darken, and sometimes thick fluid called colostrum may leak from your breasts.

All of these changes are normal.

Breast tenderness

Your breasts will **increase in size** as your milk glands enlarge and the fat tissue enlarges, causing **breast firmness** and **tenderness** typically during pregnancy's **first** and **last few months**.

Recommendations:

- Wear a bra that provides firm support.

- Choose cotton bras or those made from natural fibers.

- Get a bigger bra as your breasts become larger and fuller. Your bra should fit well without irritating your nipples. Try maternity or nursing bras, which provide more support and can be used after delivery while breastfeeding.

- Try wearing a bra during the night. Wash your breasts with warm water only. Don't use soap or other products that can cause dryness.

- As breasts prepare for lactation, they often become tender and sensitive. Wearing a supportive, well-fitting bra and using warm compresses can offer relief.

9. CONSTIPATION

Your hormones, as well as vitamins and iron supplements, pressure from the growing uterus may cause constipation (difficulty passing stool or incomplete or infrequent passage of hard stools). Pressure on your rectum from your uterus may also cause constipation.

Recommendations:

- Add more fiber (such as whole grain foods, fresh fruits, and vegetables) to your diet and maintain regular bowel habits

- Drink plenty of fluids daily (at least 6-8 glasses of water and 1-2 glasses of fruit or prune juice).

- Drink warm liquids, especially in the morning. Exercise daily, Walking for 20 minutes a day may be suggested by your doctor.

- Avoid straining when you have a bowel movement.

- Discuss the use of a laxative or stool softener with your health care provider.

- Find iron preparation that is least constipating

10. DIZZINESS (FEELING FAINT)

Dizziness can occur anytime during middle to late pregnancy.

Why it happens:

- The hormone progesterone dilates blood vessels so blood tends to pool in the legs.

- More blood is also going to your growing uterus. This can cause a drop in blood pressure, especially when changing positions -- and that can make you dizzy.

- If your blood sugar levels get too low, you may feel faint.

Recommendations:

- Move around often when standing for long periods of time.

- Lie on your left side to rest. This helps circulation throughout your body.

- Avoid sudden movements. Move slowly when standing from a sitting position.

- Eat regular, small meals throughout the day to prevent low blood sugar.

- Evaluate your haemoglobin and haematocrit

- Avoid hot environments

11. DIFFICULTY IN SLEEPING

Finding a comfortable resting position can become difficult later in pregnancy.

Recommendations:

- Don't take sleep medication.

- Try drinking warm milk at bedtime.

- Try taking a warm shower or bath before bedtime.

- Use extra pillows for support while sleeping. Lying on your side, place a pillow under your head, abdomen, behind your back and between your knees, to prevent muscle strain and help you get the rest you need

- You will probably feel better lying on your left side; this improves circulation of blood throughout your body.

Heartburn is a burning feeling that starts in the stomach and seems to rise up to the throat. During pregnancy, changing hormone levels slow down your digestive system and your uterus can crowd your stomach, pushing stomach acids upward.

Recommendations:

- Eat several small meals each day instead of three large meals.

- Eat slowly.

- Drink warm liquids.

- Avoid fried, spicy, or any foods that seem to give you indigestion.

- Don't lie down right after eating.

- Keep the head of your bed higher than the foot of your bed. Or, place pillows under your shoulders to prevent stomach acids from rising into your chest.

- Don't mix fatty foods with sweets in one meal, and try to separate liquids and solids at meals.

- Try heartburn relievers such as antacids.

13. HAEMORRHOIDS

Haemorrhoids are swollen veins that appear as painful lumps on the anus. During pregnancy, they may form as a result of increased circulation and pressure on the rectum and vagina from your growing baby.

Recommendations:

- Maintain regular bowel habits and avoid constipation, Constipation can cause haemorrhoids and will make them more painful.

- Avoid sitting or standing for long periods of time; change your position frequently.

- Don't strain during a bowel movement.

- Apply ice packs or cold compresses to the area or take a warm bath a few times a day to provide relief.

- Avoid tight-fitting underwear, pants, or panty.

- Apply topical or anesthetic ointments to area.

- If you still need more help, consult your health care provider and use prescribed stool softeners.

14. VARICOSE VEINS

Pregnancy may affect your circulation, which can enlarge or swell your legs' veins.

Recommendations:

Although varicose veins are usually hereditary , here are some preventive tips:

- Avoid standing or sitting in one place for long periods. It's important to get up and move around often.

- Avoid remaining in any position that might restrict the circulation in your legs (such as **crossing your legs while sitting**).

- Elevate your legs and feet while sitting.

- Exercise regularly

- Wear support hose but avoid any leg wear that is too tight or constraining.

- Elevate legs regularly.

15. LEG CRAMPS

Pressure from your growing uterus can cause leg cramps or sharp pains down your legs.

Recommendations:

- Be sure to eat and drink foods that are rich in calcium.

- Wear comfortable, low-heeled shoes.

- Avoid any leg wear that is too tight.

- Elevate your legs frequently, avoid crossing your legs.

- Exercise daily.

- Stretch your legs before going to bed.

- Avoid lying on your back, since the weight of your body and the pressure of your enlarged uterus can slow the circulation in your legs, causing cramps.

- Gently stretch any muscle that becomes cramped by straightening your leg, flexing your foot, and pulling your toes toward you

- Massage the cramp or apply heat or a hot water bottle to the sore area.

16. NASAL CONGESTION

You may have a stuffy nose or feel like you have a cold. Pregnancy hormones sometimes dry out the nose's lining, making it inflamed and swollen.

Recommendations:

- Apply a warm, wet wash cloth to your cheeks, eyes, and nose to reduce congestion.

- Don't use nose sprays; they can aggravate your symptoms.

- Drink plenty of fluids (at least 6-8 glasses of fluids a day) to thin mucus.

- Elevate your head with an extra pillow while sleeping to prevent mucus from blocking your throat.

- Use a humidifier or vaporizer to add moisture to the air.

- Take a warm shower or bath.

- Avoid decongestants.

- Use Normal saline drops.

17. SHORTNESS OF BREATH

Shortness of breath can happen due to increased upward pressure from the uterus.

Recommendations:

- When walking, slow down and rest a few moments.

- Raise your arms over your head (this lifts your rib cage and allows you to breathe in more air).

- Avoid lying flat on your back, and try sleeping with your head elevated.

- If prolonged shortness of breathing continues or you experience sharp pain when inhaling, contact your health care provider. You could have a pulmonary embolism (blood clot in the lungs).

18. PTYALISM (EXCESSIVE SALIVATION)

Cause Unknown

Recommendations:

- Perform frequent mouth care.

- Chew gum.

- Decrease fluid intake at night.

- Maintain fluid intake during day

19. STRETCH MARKS

- **Stretch marks are a type of scar tissue that forms when the skin's normal elasticity is not enough for the stretching that occurs during pregnancy.** They usually appear on the abdomen and can also appear on the breasts, buttocks or thighs.

- Though they won't disappear completely, stretch marks will fade after delivery. Stretch marks affect the surface under the skin and are not preventable.

Recommendations:

- Be sure that your diet contains enough sources of the nutrients needed for healthy skin (especially vitamins C and E).

- Apply lotion to your skin to keep it soft and reduce dryness.

- Exercise daily.

20. VAGINAL DISCHARGE

- Normal vaginal secretions increase during pregnancy due to greater blood supply and hormones.

- Normal vaginal discharge is white or clear, isn't irritating, is odourless, and may look yellow when dry on your underwear or panty liners.

Recommendations:

- Choose cotton underwear or brands made from natural fibers.

- Avoid tight-fitting jeans or pants.

- Do not douche. Douching can introduce air into your circulatory system or break your bag of waters in later pregnancy.

- Clean the vaginal area often with soap and water.

- Wipe yourself from front to back.

- Contact your health care provider if you have **burning, itching, irritation or swelling, bad odour, bloody discharge, or bright yellow or green discharge** (these symptoms could be a **sign of infection**).

21. BACKACHES

Backaches are usually caused by the strain put on the back muscles, **changing hormone levels, and changes in your posture.**

Recommendations:

- Wear low-heeled (but not flat) shoes.

- Avoid lifting heavy objects.

- Squat down with your knees bent when picking things up instead of bending down at the waist.

- Don't stand on your feet for long periods. If you need to stand for long periods, place one foot on a stool or box for support.

- Sit in a chair with good back support, or place a small pillow behind your lower back. Also, place your feet on a footrest or stool.

- Check that your bed is firm. If needed, put a board between the mattress and box spring.

- Sleep on your left or right side with a pillow between your legs for support.

- Apply a hot water bottle, heating pad on low setting, take a warm bath or shower, or try massage.

- Perform exercises, as advised by your health care provider, to make your back muscles stronger and help relieve the soreness.

- Maintain good posture. Standing up straight will ease the strain on your back.

- Contact your health care provider if you have a low backache that goes around your stomach and does not subside within one hour after you change position or rest. This might be a sign of premature labour.

- Walk with pelvis tilted forward.

- Perform pelvic rocking or tilting

22. ABDOMINAL PAIN OR DISCOMFORT

Sharp, shooting pains on either side of your stomach may result from the stretching the tissue supporting your growing uterus. These pains may also travel down your thigh and into your leg.

Recommendations:

- Change your position or activity until you are comfortable; avoid sharp turns or movements.

- If you have a sudden pain in your abdomen, bend forward to the point of pain to relieve tension and relax the tissue.

- Apply a hot water bottle, heating pad, or take a warm bath or shower.

- Try a massage.

- Make sure you are getting enough fluids.

- Take Tylenol (acetaminophen) occasionally.

- Contact your health care provider if the pain is severe or constant or if you are less than 36 weeks pregnant and you have signs of labor.

23. BRAXTON-HICKS CONTRACTIONS

The uterine muscles will contract (tighten) starting as early as the second trimester of pregnancy on. Irregular, infrequent contractions are called

Braxton-Hicks contractions (also known as **"false labor pains"**). These are normal during pregnancy.

Recommendations:

Try to relax -Change positions. Sometimes this can ease the contractions.

Navigating these discomforts involves a combination of **lifestyle adjustments, self-care practices,** and, when needed, **guidance from healthcare professionals.**

Embracing a holistic approach to managing physical discomforts during pregnancy can contribute to a more comfortable and fulfilling journey towards motherhood.

Danger signs of pregnancy

- Vaginal bleeding including spotting

- Persistent abdominal pain

- Severe and Persistent vomiting

- Sudden gush of fluid through vagina

- Absence or decreased foetal movement

- Severe head ache

- Oedema of hands, face, legs & feet

- Fever above 100 F(Greater than 37.7 degrees C)

- Digginess, blurred vision, double vision.

- Painful urination

CHAPTER: 13

NUTRITION AND LIFE STYLE DURING PREGNANCY

A healthy diet and lifestyle helps you to keep well during pregnancy and gives your baby the best possible start in life.

What should you eat?

- A healthy diet is very important if you are pregnant or trying to get pregnant. Make sure that you **eat a variety of different foods every day** in order to get the **right balance of nutrients** that you and your baby need. You should also **avoid certain foods.**

- You will probably find that you are more hungry than normal, but you **don't need to 'Eat for two'** – even if you are expecting twins or triplets.

- **Have breakfast every day**. This will help you to avoid snacking on foods that are high in fat and sugar.

FRUIT AND VEGETABLES

- Fruit and vegetables provide   vitamins and minerals and   fibre, which helps digestion and prevents constipation.

- Don't over -cook them.

POTATOES, BREAD, RICE, PASTA AND OTHER STARCHY CARBOHYDRATES

- Carbohydrates are satisfying without containing too many calories, and are an important source of vitamins and fibre.

- They include bread, potatoes, breakfast cereals, pasta, rice, oats, noodles, maize, millet, yams, cornmeal and sweet potatoes.

- These foods should be the main part of every meal. **Eat whole grain varieties** when you can as these add **extra fibre** to our diet.

FOODS HIGH IN FAT, SALT AND SUGARS

This includes products such as **chocolate, cakes, biscuits, full-sugar soft drinks, butter and ice-cream.**

As these foods are not needed in the diet, try to limit their consumption.

Avoid foods which are high in fat, salt and sugar!

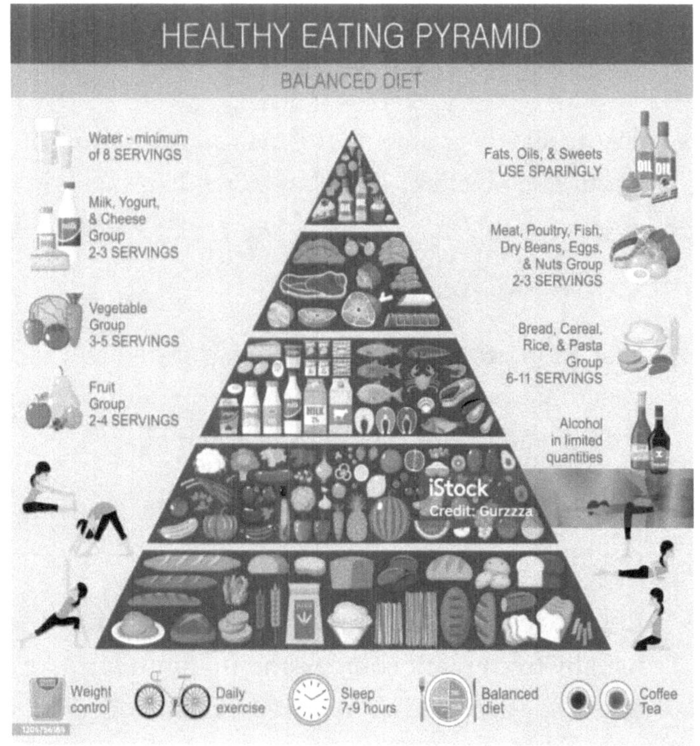

BEANS, PULSES, FISH, EGGS, MEAT AND OTHER PROTEINS

- Good sources of protein include beans, pulses, fish, eggs and meat. These foods are also good sources of essential vitamins and minerals. Eat moderate amounts each day.

- Choose lean meat, remove the skin from poultry and cook using only a little fat.

- You should try to limit the amount of red meat or processed meat

- Make sure poultry, pork, burgers and sausages are cooked all the way through.

- Try to eat two portions of fish a week, one of which should be oily fish. There are some fish that you should avoid.

OILS AND SPREADS

- This food group includes all unsaturated oils including vegetable oil, rapeseed oil, olive oil sunflower oil and soft spreads made from unsaturated oils.

- Butters should be eaten less often and in small amounts.

- **Unsaturated fats are healthier fats** that are usually from plant sources and in liquid form as oil, for example vegetable oil, rapeseed oil and olive oil. Using

- Remember that all types of fat are high in energy and should be limited in the diet.

DAIRY AND ALTERNATIVES

- Milk and dairy foods like cheese, soya drinks and yogurts are important because they contain protein, calcium and other nutrients that your baby needs.

- Eat two or three portions a day, using low-fat varieties, for example, semi-skimmed or skimmed milk, low-fat yogurt and half-fat hard cheese.

- Aim to drink 6-8 glasses of fluid every day. Water, lower fat milk and sugar-free drinks including tea and coffee all count..

FOODS TO AVOID

There are some foods that you should not eat when you are pregnant because they may make you ill or harm your baby.

You should avoid:

- Some types of cheese.

- Raw or undercooked meat

- Liver products.

- Supplements containing vitamin A.

  Don't take high-dose multivitamin supplements, fish liver oil supplements or any supplements containing vitamin A.

- Some types of fish.

- Don't eat shark, marlin and swordfish, and limit the amount of tuna you eat as they contain high levels of mercury, which can damage your baby's developing nervous system.

- Unpasteurised milk

Eating a healthy, varied diet will help you to get the vitamins and minerals you need while you are pregnant. However some vitamins and minerals that are especially important include:

Folic acid.

- Folic acid is important as it can reduce the risk of neural tube defects such as spina bifida in your unborn child. If you are thinking about getting pregnant, you should take a 400 microgram folic acid tablet every day until you are 12 weeks pregnant.

- You should also eat foods that contain folic acid, such as **green leafy vegetables, fortified breakfast cereals** and **brown rice**.

- Some **breakfast cereals, breads** and **margarines** have folic acid added to them.

Iodine supplements

- There is no current recommendation in some regions to take iodine supplements during pregnancy, and you should be able to get all the iodine you need by eating a varied diet.

- If you do choose to take iodine supplements, do not take more than 0.5 milligramsa day, as this could be harmful.

Vitamin D.

- All pregnant women should take 10 microgram supplement of vitamin D during autumn and winter months as sunlight is not strong enough to make vitamin D during this time (October to the end of March).

- You need vitamin D to keep your bones healthy and to provide your baby with enough vitamin D for the first few months of their life. Vitamin D regulates the amount of calcium and phosphate in the body, and these are needed to help keep bones and teeth healthy.

- The best source of vitamin D is summer sunlight. The amount of time you need in the sun to make enough vitamin D is different for every person and depends on things like skin type, time of day and time of the year but you don't need to sunbathe. Deficiency of vitamin D can cause children's bones to soften and can lead to rickets.

- Only a few foods contain vitamin D, including **oily fish like sardines, fortified margarines, some breakfast cereals and eggs.**

Iron.

- If you are low in iron, you will probably get very tired and you can become anaemic. **Lean meat, green, leafy vegetables, dried fruit and nuts all contain iron.**

- Many breakfast cereals have iron added.

  - Iron supplements are available as tablets or a liquid

Vitamin C.

- Vitamin C helps your body absorb iron. Citrus fruits, tomatoes, broccoli, peppers, blackcurrants, potatoes and some pure fruit juices are good sourcesof vitamin C.

- If your iron levels are low, it may help to drink orange juice with an iron-rich meal.

Calcium

- Calcium is vital for making your baby's bones and teeth.

- Dairy products and fish with edible bones like sardines are rich in calcium. Breakfast cereals, dried fruit such as figs and apricots, bread, almonds, tofu (a vegetable protein made from soya beans) and green leafy vegetables like watercress, broccoli and curly kale are other good sources of calcium.

LIFESTYLE

HYGIENE

- Daily bath and all over wash -stimulating, refreshing and relaxing

- Hot bath to be avoided,-may cause fainting and fatigue.

- Regular washing of genital area, axillae and breasts - because of increased sweat and discharge

- **Avoid Vaginal douches**-Douching leads to the spread of an infection or even the development of an infection by altering the balance of normal bacteria present in the vagina,

BREAST CARE

Wear right bra- Always remember to wear the right sized bra to avoid suffocation and discomfort. Avoid tight bras and bras with underwire.

Massage- Massaging the breasts with coconut oil can also aid in blood circulation.

No Soap on the Nipple- Always ensure not to use any soap on the nipple during your daily baths. Soap tends to dry out the nipples and it can lead to cracking of the nipple area.

Moisturizing Creams- After bath apply some moisturizing cream on the nipples if they feel too dry.

Nipple protector- get some nipple protectors to prevent the soreness from being aggravated.

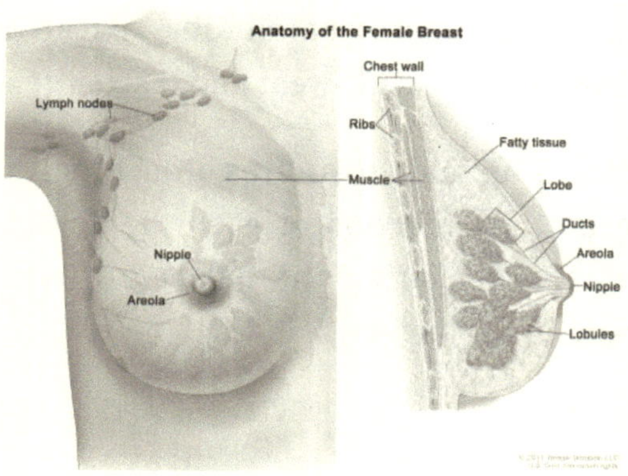

DENTAL CARE

- Brush your teeth carefully in the morning, before going to bed and after every meal

- See your Dentist regularly for routine examination and cleaning

- Tooth extraction if needed to be done only under local anaesthesia

- Gum problems during pregnancy could lead to preterm, low birth weight babies

- Increased hormone levels during pregnancy will worsen dental problems.

- Avoid self - medication for dental pain, this can affect your child

- Dental procedures are safe during 4-6 months of pregnancy

Have a dental check- up during and after pregnancy

DRESS AND SHOE DURING PREGNANCY

- Avoid tight dresses and constricting bands on the legs

- Use loose , light cotton clothing

- Wear moderate to low heeled or flat shoe to minimize pelvic tilt and backache

TRAVEL

Avoid unnecessary travel throughout pregnancy, especially in the first trimester to avoid bleeding and abortion and Third trimester to avoid premature labor

- If travelling is inevitable, travel by train or flight and avoid road travel.

SEXUAL ACTIVITY

Avoid sex during 1st **trimester** and **last 6 weeks of pregnancy** and **throughout pregnancy** if there is **H/O a previous abortion**

ALCOHOL

- The risk of damage to your baby's physical and mental development increases the more you drink which is why binge drinking is especially harmful.

- This risk relates to a range of conditions including **Foetal Alcohol Syndrome (FAS)** and **Foetal Alcohol Spectrum Disorder (FASD).**

SMOKING

- Every cigarette you smoke harms your baby. Cigarettes restrict the essential oxygen supply to your baby. So their tiny heart has to beat harder every time you smoke.

- Cigarettes contain over 4,000 chemicals. Protecting your baby from tobacco smoke is one of the best things you can do to give your child a healthy start in life.

If you stop smoking:

- You are more likely to have a healthier pregnancy and a healthier baby.

- You will reduce the risk of stillbirth. Underweight babies, premature births

- Babies of mothers who smoke are, on average, 200g (about 8oz) lighter than other babies, may have problems during and after labour and are more prone to infection.

- You will reduce the risk of sudden infant death, also known as 'cot death'.

Second hand smoke

- If your partner or anyone else who lives with you smokes, it can affect you and your baby both before and after birth. You may also find it more difficult to quit.

- Second hand smoke can cause low birth weight and sudden infant death.

PILLS, MEDICINES AND OTHER DRUGS

Some **medicines,** including some common **painkillers, can harm your baby's health,**

Use as few over the counter medicines as possible.

Medicines and treatments that are usually safe include **paracetamol, most antibiotics, dental treatments** (including local anaesthetics), some **immunisations** (including **tetanus, pertussis and flu**)

Make sure the medicine is safe to take when pregnant.

ILLEGAL DRUGS

Illegal drugs like cannabis, ecstasy, cocaine and heroin can harm your baby. If you use any illegal drugs, it is important to talk to your doctor or midwife so that they can provide you with advice and support to help you stop.

They can also refer you for additional support. Some dependent drug users initially need drug treatment to stabilise or come off drugs to keep the baby safe.

X-RAYS

X-rays should be avoided in pregnancy if possible. Make sure that your dentist knows you are pregnant.

- It is recommended that if you are thinking of having a baby, your BMI should be between 20 and 25.

- If you are overweight, ie **BMI of over 25** you should aim to lose weight before becoming pregnant.

- Being **obese (having a BMI greater than 30)** during pregnancy can put you at increased risk of pregnancy complications such as **gestational diabetes** and **thromboembolism.** Therefore if you are planning a pregnancy speak to a health professional about achieving a healthy weight.

- It can be dangerous for your baby too, causing **premature birth, birth defects, miscarriage** and **stillbirth.**

- BMI is a calculation that health professionals use to work out whether a person is a healthy weight. It is **calculated by weight in kilograms divided by height in meters squared.**

EXERCISE

Keeping active

- The more active and fit you are during pregnancy, the easier it will be for you to adapt to your changing shape and weight gain. It will also help you to cope with labour and to get back into shape after the birth.

- Keep up your normal daily physical activity or exercise (sport, dancing or just walking to the shops and back) for as long as you feel comfortable.

- Don't exhaust yourself, and remember that you may need to slow down as your pregnancy progresses or if your doctor advises you to.

- 150 minutes of moderate physical activity spread throughout the week is recommended in pregnancy or half an hour of walking each day can be enough.

- Avoid any strenuous exercise in hot weather.

- Drink plenty of water and other fluids.

CHAPTER: 14

SELF - CARE DURING PREGNANCY

Nurturing the Miracle Within: Self-Care During Pregnancy

Welcoming a new life into the world is a magical and transformative journey, but it also demands special attention to self-care during pregnancy. This chapter is your ultimate guide to navigating this incredible period of your life with grace, ensuring both your physical and emotional well-being. Let's embark on this journey together, discovering the art of self-care that will nurture both you and the miracle growing within.

Nourishing your body: A symphony of nutrients

During pregnancy, your body requires an array of essential nutrients to support the development of your baby. Explore the power of a well-balanced diet, incorporating key nutrients such as folic acid, iron, and calcium. Learn about delicious and nutritious meals that not only satiate your cravings but also promote optimal fetal growth.

GENTLE EXERCISES FOR MOM AND BABY

Discover the benefits of staying active during pregnancy through safe and gentle exercises. From prenatal yoga to low-impact workouts, find a routine that suits your body's needs and promotes a healthy pregnancy. Exercise not only boosts your physical well-being but also enhances your mood and prepares your body for labor.

Pampering your changing body:

Embrace the changes your body undergoes during pregnancy with love and care. Explore beauty and skincare routines that prioritize natural ingredients, promoting healthy skin while addressing common concerns like stretch marks and swelling. Treat yourself to soothing massages and baths that provide relaxation and relief.

EMOTIONAL WELLBEING

Mindfullness and bonding

Embrace the changes your body undergoes during pregnancy with love and care. Explore beauty and skincare routines that prioritize natural ingredients, promoting healthy skin while addressing common concerns like stretch marks and swelling. Treat yourself to soothing massages and baths that provide relaxation and relief.

Communicating with your partner

Pregnancy is a journey shared not only by you but also by your partner. Learn effective communication strategies to navigate the emotional highs and lows together. Discover ways to strengthen your relationship, ensuring a supportive and harmonious environment for both of you as you prepare to become parents.

Seeking community support

Build a network of support that includes friends, family, and fellow expectant mothers. Share experiences, seek advice, and create a supportive community that understands the unique challenges and joys of pregnancy.

Surround yourself with positivity and encouragement as you embark on this transformative chapter of your life.

As you embark on this incredible journey of pregnancy, remember that **self-care** is not a luxury but a necessity. Nurturing your physical and emotional well-being is not only beneficial for you but also crucial for the health and development of your baby.

Embrace the art of self-care, savoring every moment as you prepare to welcome the miracle within.

DISCLAIMER

The information provided in this book, "Celebrate Pain-Free Periods," is intended for general informational purposes only. While the book discusses various methods and medicines that may contribute to a pain-free menstrual experience, it is important to note that individual circumstances may vary.

Readers are strongly advised to consult their Health Care Provider before initiating any new medication or treatment regimen, especially if they have pre-existing medical conditions, are currently taking prescribed medications, or are pregnant or breastfeeding. The author and publisher are not responsible for any adverse effects or consequences resulting from the use of the information provided in this book. It is crucial to seek personalized medical advice to ensure the safest and most effective course of action for your specific situation.

Always prioritize your well-being and consult a qualified healthcare professional for tailored advice.

ABOUT THE AUTHOR

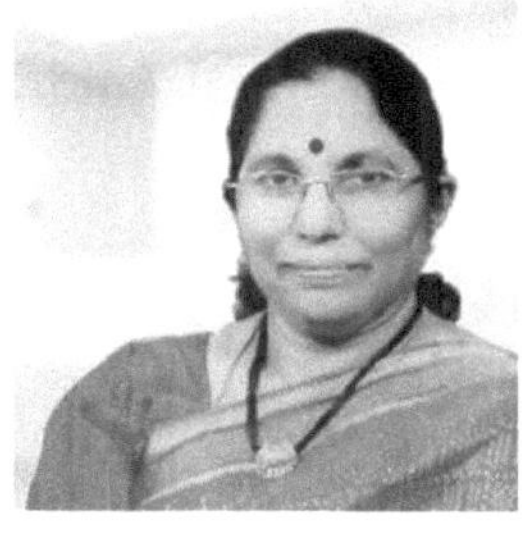

Dr. Vijayalakshmi Aluri is a prolific and highly accomplished writer whose literary achievements have left an indelible mark on the world of literature. With a diverse repertoire that spans across various genres, she has captivated readers with her talent and insightful storytelling.

As the author of around 150 captivating short stories, she has a unique ability to weave intricate narratives that resonate deeply with readers.

Her stories have garnered recognition and accolades, winning prestigious prizes conducted by different magazines. These tales have been broadcasted by All India Radio, reaching a wider audience and leaving a lasting impact on listeners.

Dr. Aluri's literary prowess extends beyond the realm of fiction. She has penned four thought-provoking novels that delve into the depths of the human experience, offering profound insights into our collective journey.

Her ability to effortlessly blend realism and imagination creates a tapestry of emotions that keeps readers enthralled from start to finish.

Not content with her already impressive contributions to literature, Dr. Aluri has also made significant strides in the field of health education. Her books, such as "Matrutvam" and "Adolescent girls' health," serve as essential guides for individuals navigating various stages of life.

Additionally, her translation work has brought world-famous health education books to the Telugu-speaking community, making crucial knowledge accessible to all.

Dr. Vijayalakshmi Aluri's dedication to promoting health education and empowering individuals is evident in the distribution of 100,000 copies of "Adolescent girls' health" to schools and organizations. Her tireless efforts, backed by the support of government and non-government organizations, have had a profound impact on the lives of countless young girls.

Recognized for her literary contributions, Dr. Aluri's name holds a prominent place in esteemed publications such as the "Who is who of Indian writers" and the "Who is Who of Indian Translators." Her work has been included in textbooks and academic curricula, cementing her legacy as a writer whose words have shaped the intellectual landscape.

Dr. Vijayalakshmi Aluri's passion for literature, combined with her commitment to promoting health education, has touched the hearts and minds of readers worldwide.

Her stories and books have the power to inspire, educate, and transform lives, making her an author whose literary legacy will endure for generations to come.

In addition to her remarkable literary achievements, Dr. Vijayalakshmi Aluri has expanded her reach through self-publishing on Amazon. With an entrepreneurial spirit, she has independently released two captivating fiction books, "The War" and "Battlefield."

These works showcase her talent for crafting engaging narratives that transport readers into immersive worlds filled with suspense, emotion, and profound insights.

Furthermore, Dr. Aluri's commitment to health education shines through in her self-published book, "Celebrate Your Adolescence." This empowering guide provides invaluable information and guidance to adolescents, encouraging them to embrace the transformative journey of adolescence with confidence, self-awareness, and a celebration of their unique selves.

Continuing her dedication to educating and empowering individuals, Dr. Aluri is set to release another significant health education book, "Celebrate Your Menses," which will be available on Amazon.

This forthcoming publication promises to be a ground breaking resource, shedding light on a crucial and often misunderstood aspect of a woman's life. Dr. Aluri's compassionate and informative approach will provide readers with the knowledge and tools to navigate this natural and important phase of their lives.

By self-publishing on Amazon, Dr. Vijayalakshmi Aluri has embraced the opportunities presented by the digital age, ensuring that her important messages and stories reach a global audience.

Her books, both fiction and health education, exemplify her commitment to empowering individuals, fostering understanding, and inspiring personal growth. With each publication, she continues to leave an indelible impact on readers, establishing herself as a versatile and influential author in the literary world.

MAY I REQUEST YOU FOR A SMALL FAVOUR?

At the outset, a big **Thank you** for taking your valuable time to read my book. I hope that you received some practical insights that will impact your life positively.

I highly appreciate your generous gesture of choosing my book among thousands of books that are published each and every day.

May I have few more seconds of your productive time?

I would love to have your precious review on my book. Reviews might not matter for big name writers, but they are of extreme help for new authors like me who don't have much following.

I highly appreciate if you could leave a review of the book. As you know, reviews are the life line of any author. I humbly appeal to you to provide a review on the store you purchased this book from. I feel honoured to have your exquisite review.

BOOKS BY THIS AUTHOR

1) THE WAR

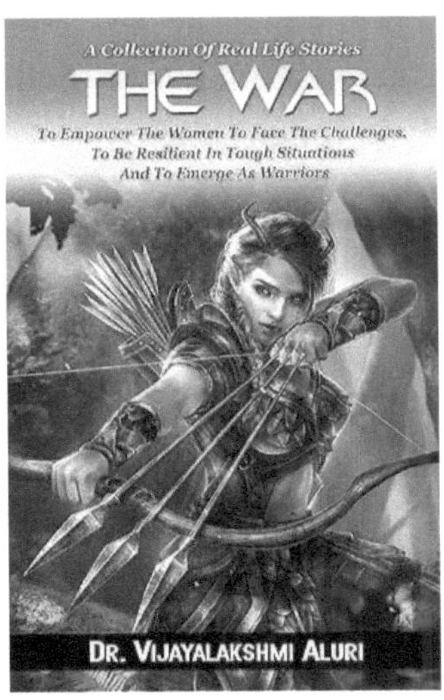

A Collection Of Real Life Stories To Empower The Women To Face The Challenges, To Be Resilient In Tough Situations And To Emerge As Warriors

The War is a compilation of 7 stories projecting the different issues propelling the lives of people and providing insights into women's struggles to empower themselves in the present-day socio-cultural scenario.

Women, anywhere in the world are subjected to disrespect, inequality, injustice, exploitation, endless abuse, gender discrimination, gender pay gap, gender violence etc., more so in India, a country where women are given the status of a goddess.

The War inspires the people to let their hearts be filled with empathy in the unprecedented calamities like Covid pandemic. It reflects the plight of health care personnel working in the most vulnerable conditions, yet preserving the human feel. It mentions the existing inequalities exposed by Lock down and inspires the people to have humane relationships with others, especially in tough times.

'Flower Garden' emphasizes the importance of nurturing human values. The story declares that though money is the pivotal element in our lives, there are many vital components of human life which are more precious than money. It also affirms that no person should die because of non-availability of healthcare at right time. (This story was selected as one of the best 12 stories out of around 1400 stories translated into English from almost all Indian languages, by Humanscape, a magazine from Mumbai)

'Break the shackles' represents the life of educated and earning women surrounded by the shackles of patriarchy and their struggles to overcome the hurdles. While men can enjoy both the secure family and a career, women face many visible and invisible roadblocks to have them. They would be threatened emotionally and culturally to opt for any one of them. It questions patriarchal society which denies the women the right to have autonomy and decision making power.

'Quagmire' questions the systems which allow the mafia gangs to make the drugs as easily available as chocolates in the colleges, schools and universities, leading to the destruction of future of the youth. It criticizes the apathy of the citizens and society at large when systems fail to control the evils of society. It also gives a lucid picture of the innocent youth drowning in the quagmire of addictions.

'The Path' shows a path to the present-day youth to become responsible and productive citizens of the country protecting themselves from becoming prey to the newly emerging vices in modern life..

'Burning furnace' gives a bird's eye view of the impact of globalization and its offshoot, new economic reforms encouraging special economic zones, huge big dams etc, driving the common people away from their lands, their villages and their livelihoods. It questions the unjust policies of the Governments, which should have an obligation to protect the people. The story also questions the development model in which the fruits of development do not trickle down to the poor and widens the gap between the powerful rich and the powerless poor.

'Fragrance' portrays the struggle of a resilient woman, who was forced to leave her village to escape from hunger, depression and violence from her husband and toil in the city to bring up her children. After reading these stories, you will have a vivid picture of the sentiments, emotions, valor, perseverance, hopes, aspirations and goals of people, especially women, apart from their struggles, sufferings and sacrifices in a traditional socio-cultural setting.

All the stories have a common ideology, **"Humankind is my business"**

Read, enjoy and join in this most beautiful business to transform this world happier

Please scan the below QR code to buy and read it from Amazon:

2) BATTLEFIELD

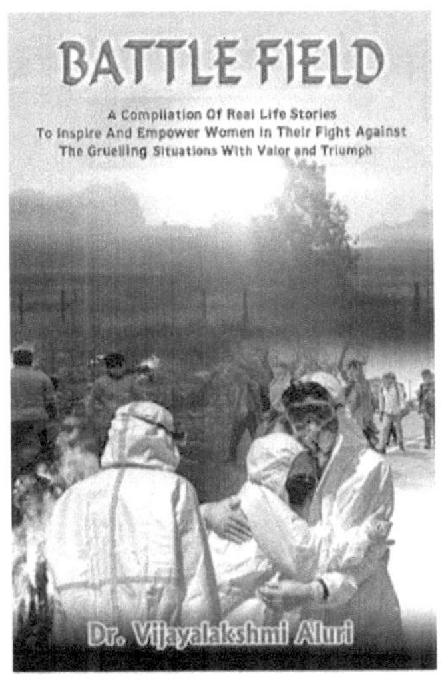

A Compilation Of Real Life Stories To Inspire and Empower Women In Their Fight Against Gruelling Situations With Valor And Triumph

Are you fed up of reading mere imaginative and mock stories?

Are You Passionate To Have A Fresh Experience Of The Intense True Stories With Different Dimensions Of Life?

Do you want To read the stories of women who are victims of poverty and patriarchy?

Do you want to get inspired by the Empowered and Courageous women who stood up against all odds?

Then proceed To Read these real life stories These poignant stories, from the pen of a compassionate doctor, hold a mirror to present-day society.

The stories deal with themes ranging from incest to the trials and tribulations faced by the voiceless underprivileged to the present day horrifying situation the world is in, due to the epidemic, and particularly the alarming medical crisis our country is faced with.

Despite the horrifying circumstances which could plunge any person into the depths of despair, the resilience, tenacity and strength of character displayed by the protagonist of **"The Inferno",** one of the stories, is no less than a beacon of light and an inspiration to the many unfortunate women.

Yet another story portrays the plight of the unlettered voiceless and disadvantaged people bringing to light the inequitable society we live in.

The story, **"Battlefield",** provides readers with a gallery view of the happenings occurring at a frenetic pace in a hospital.

Furthermore, the practical problems faced by the Frontline workers, tasked with handling Covid cases, is shown from a human perspective.

Please scan the below QR code to buy from Amazon:

Scan me!

3) CELEBRATE YOUR ADOLESCENCE

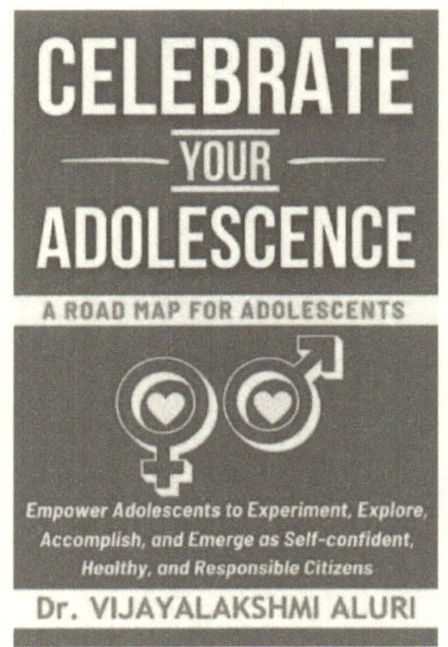

Did you ever questioned yourself:

Am I Normal?

Am I a child or an adult?

Have you ever wondered why there are changes in your body?

Did the changes make you feel embarrassed, scared or ashamed?

Were you ever overwhelmed while experiencing the physical, psychological, emotional, sexual and social changes, all simultaneously?

Rapid growth... Cause of Concern!

Do you want to have a smooth, safe, healthy, happy and productive adolescence?

Then this book, **"Celebrate your Adolescence"** is for you.

Do you want to support your adolescent child to pass through this crucial phase of transition without the impact of myths, misconceptions and misinformation that lead to life-long consequences?

Do you want to guide your student to travel through the right path to attain holistic development through knowledge and achieve their full potential to emerge as productive and responsible citizens?

Here is a book,

A **torch** to throw light on the various challenges and opportunities adolescents encounter in this crucial phase of their lives.

A **resource** to provide authentic knowledge for Adolescents, enabling them to make well- informed choices.

A **tool** that can help build systems and processes to strengthen and promote the positive health of adolescents.

This book gives you clear insights of Adolescence

Please scan the below QR code to buy from Amazon:

Scan me!

4) CELEBRATE YOUR MENSES

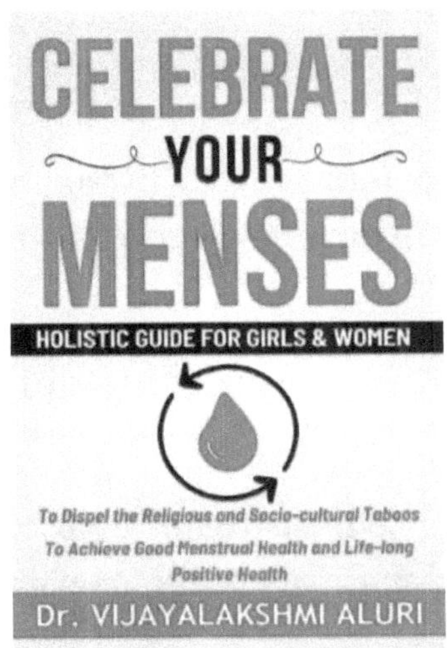

Are you excited to get your period or a bit frightened?

Let your fears be calmed and Let your anxious questions be answered with this book, **Celebrate Your Menses**, an **arc lamp** which dispels the darkness of myths and misconceptions surrounding monthly periods.

"Celebrate Your Menses" offers a comprehensive guide to menstruation, focusing on the physical, emotional, and spiritual aspects of the menstrual cycle.

Menstruation is a natural process that every woman experiences, yet it's often stigmatized and shrouded in **shame** and **secrecy. It's time to change that**.

From a young age, girls are taught to hide their pads and tampons and to avoid talking about their periods in public.

This culture of shame and secrecy can have profound effects on how they view their bodies and themselves.

But what if we could change that?

What if we could learn to celebrate our menstrual cycle and view it as a powerful force for good in our lives?

"Celebrate Your Menses." is a powerful tool to achieve this goal.

This book is not just for those who menstruate but also for anyone who wants to understand more about the menstrual cycle and how it impacts our lives.

Whether you're a teenager just starting to menstruate or an adult navigating perimenopause, this book will provide you with valuable insights and tools to make your menstrual cycle a positive and empowering experience.

This book will explore the **science** behind menstruation, **demystify common myths and misconceptions**, and offer **practical tips for managing symptoms and discomfort**.

It will also delve into the **cultural and historical significance of menstruation**, from ancient traditions and rituals to modern-day menstrual activism.

"Celebrate Your Menses" reflects the need for a celebration of the female body and the incredible power it holds and offers tips for harnessing that power to improve the lives of girls and women. It also explores how menstruation impacts the physical, emotional, and spiritual health of girls and women.

The book is divided into different chapters, each of which covers a different aspect of menstruation, **physical aspects of menstruation**, including an overview of the menstrual cycle; emotional, psychological, social and spiritual aspects of menstruation; Menstrual products, beliefs, myths, misconceptions, taboos and stigmas surrounding menstruation and how they impact negatively on women's health and disempower women; the importance of menstrual hygiene and its positive impacts.

Throughout the book, the author emphasizes **the importance of celebrating menstruation and embracing it as a natural and essential part of a woman's life.**

She encourages women to view **their menstrual cycle as a source of strength and empowerment,** rather than **something to be ashamed of or hidden**.

At its core, **"Celebrate Your Menses"** is a call to action for women to reclaim their menstrual cycle, view it as a positive and empowering force in their lives and celebrate the incredible power, wisdom and transformation of their bodies.

Let's break the silence and start a conversation about menstruation that is positive, inclusive, and empowering.

By breaking the silence around menstruation and celebrating our bodies, we can create a more just and equitable world for women.

So let's get started - **it's time to celebrate your menses!**

Please scan the below QR code to buy from Amazon:

Scan Me

5) CELEBRATE PAIN-FREE PERIODS

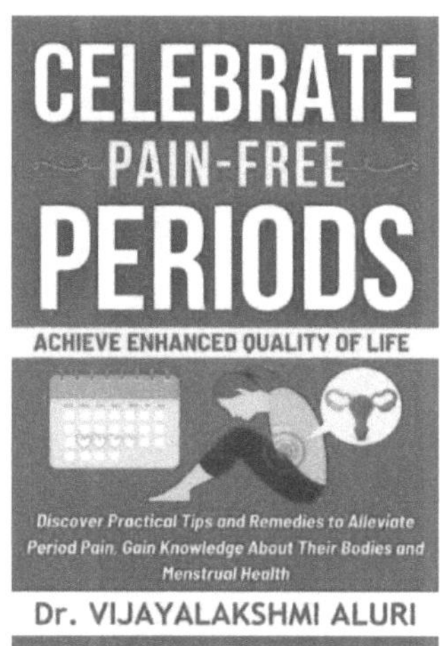

WHY TO READ THIS BOOK?

Celebrate Pain-Free Periods is a comprehensive exploration of the complex and often misunderstood world of menstruation, including its associated myths, taboos, and stigmas.

This book delves deep into the physical and emotional aspects of menstruation, shedding light on conditions like PMS, PMDD, and Dysmenorrhea while also addressing societal beliefs & misconceptions surrounding menstruation.

With insightful chapters and enlightening stories, this book aims to **educate, empower, and break the silence surrounding menstruation.**

Celebrate Pain-Free Periods is a comprehensive guide that delves deep into the intricacies of the menstrual cycle, offering insights, solutions, and empowerment to help women achieve a healthier, happier relationship with their bodies.

The book begins by laying a strong foundation of knowledge about the menstrual cycle. It explains the phases of the cycle, the hormonal changes that drive it, and why these changes are essential for reproduction.

With this understanding, readers gain a newfound appreciation for their bodies and the incredible mechanisms that make it all happen.

Please scan the below QR code to buy from Amazon:

SCAN ME

6) CELEBRATE TROUBLE FREE PERIODS

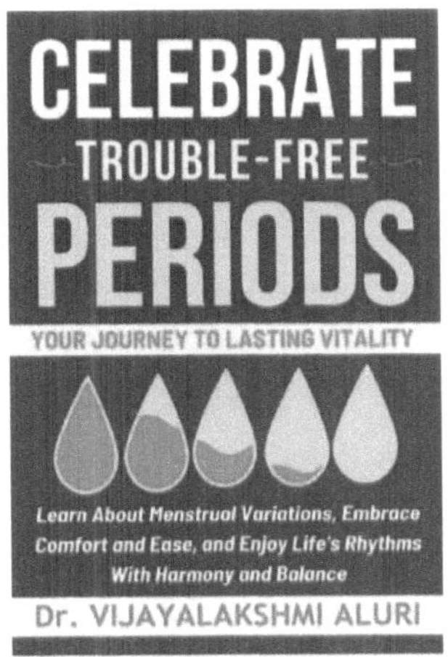

WHY TO READ THIS BOOK?

To Unlock Harmony and To Have Seamless, Stress-free periods.

To experience periods that flow coherently, free from the anxiety of irregularity and the discomfort of surprises.

To reclaim control over your menstrual cycles and To empower you to embrace each month with confidence and ease.

This comprehensive guide "Celebrate Trouble-free Periods" unravels the mysteries of menstrual irregularities, offering holistic approaches to harmonize your cycle.

It's not just about managing your periods; it's about fostering a harmonious relationship with your body, fostering well-being, and unlocking a sense of empowerment. Chapter by chapter, this book delves into a wealth of knowledge that's not only informative but engaging and empowering:

1. Understanding your cycle: Step into the world of menstrual health, demystifying the intricacies of your body's natural rhythm. Gain insights into the science behind menstrual cycles, decoding irregularities, and recognizing signs your body communicates.

2. Embracing hormonal balance: Explore the impact of hormones on your cycle and learn practical ways to maintain hormonal equilibrium. Dive into lifestyle changes, nutrition tips, and stress-reduction techniques that support hormone harmony.

3. Navigating irregularities: Uncover the reasons behind irregular periods and discover solutions tailored to your needs. Whether it's Polycystic Ovary Syndrome (PCOS), thyroid imbalances, or lifestyle factors, find guidance to navigate and manage these challenges.

4. Empowering self-care: Elevate your well-being with self-care practices that complement your menstrual health journey. From mindfulness exercises to nurturing self-compassion, these strategies will uplift your mind, body, and soul.

5. Fertility and Family planning: For those embarking on a family journey, this section delves into understanding fertility, optimizing your chances of conception, and embracing the role of a healthy cycle in family planning.

6. Elevating your life style: Elevate your lifestyle with tailored diet recommendations, exercise routines, and sleep hygiene practices that harmonize with your menstrual cycle, promoting overall health and vitality.

7. Breaking the taboos: Shatter societal taboos surrounding menstruation. Empower yourself with knowledge and confidence, fostering open conversations and changing perceptions about periods.

Embark on a transformative odyssey, armed with evidence-based insights and practical strategies. **"Celebrate Trouble-free Periods"** isn't just a book; it's your companion on a journey towards **reclaiming control, fostering self-care, and embracing the beauty of a trouble-free cycle.**

Join a community of empowered individuals, shedding the stigma around periods, and embracing menstrual health as an integral part of overall well-being. Let this guide be your beacon, leading you towards seamless, stress-free periods, and a harmonious connection with your body.

Join us on a transformative journey into the realm of trouble-free periods—an exploration that transcends irregularities, celebrates balance, and empowers individuals through harmonious cycles.

Spread the buzz that this guide should reach each and every girl before she attains menarche, so that she handles her menstrual health with knowledge and courage.

Scan Me